Dreaming a Lighthouse

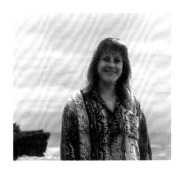

Dreaming a Lighthouse

A creative partnership –
a teenager, her doctor & cancer

Dr Hetty Rodenburg

To Anne
with love,
Hetty

STEELE ROBERTS
AOTEAROA NEW ZEALAND

All art, poems, and handwritten diary excerpts are by Wendy Potter. The front cover lighthouse photo is by Janet Potter. Photos of the seasons are by Anna Comrie-Thomson (please note, they relate to the 'seasons' or stages of Wendy's journey, not the calendar). Family photos are courtesy of the Potter family, and other photos are by Hetty Rodenburg unless otherwise credited.

National Library of New Zealand Cataloguing-in-Publication Data
Rodenburg, Hetty, 1937-
Dreaming a lighthouse : a creative partnership : a teenager, her doctor & cancer /
text Hetty Rodenburg ; all art, poems, and handwritten diary excerpts are by Wendy Potter.
ISBN 978-1-877448-84-3
1. Potter, Wendy, 1977- —Health. II. Cancer in adolescence—Patients—New Zealand
Biography.
I. Title. II. Potter, Wendy, 1977-
362.1969940092—dc 22

STEELE ROBERTS PUBLISHERS
Box 9321 Wellington, Aotearoa New Zealand
info@steeleroberts.co.nz • www.steeleroberts.co.nz

Contents

to my grandchildren, Ciara & Dylan,
who are a gift of joy

Acknowledgements

I HAVE BEEN FORTUNATE to receive help and guidance from many talented people, and want to express my heartfelt appreciation.

To Wendy's family: Janet, Cyril, Rachel and Lisa, thank you for your permission to write Wendy's story. Thank you, Lisa, for allowing me to use excerpts from your manuscript, 'Many Rivers to Cross'.

Janet, without your advice and support this book could not have been written.

Thanks to Margi Martin for inviting me to present Wendy's story at Victoria University, creating a space where I acquired valuable insights; to Lorae Parry, who with patience and humour transformed my Dutch/English into acceptable grammar; to Julie Hoyle for being a consistent inspiration since 2001; and to Raven Plaisted for laughter and nurturing throughout this expedition.

Ellie Smith, Vivienne Plumb, Sharon Crosbie, Rod MacLeod, Sarah Taylor and Pinky Agnew read the manuscript and gave valuable, constructive feedback.

Liese Groot-Alberts, Alayne Cullen, Sue Marsden, Evelyn Skinner, Stacey O'Neill, Sue Lennox, Merrilyn Moonen, Mary-Lou McCombie, Paddy Dunford and Gill Greer have been wonderful, encouraging friends.

Thanks to Moira Aberdeen for hours of transcribing; to Gerald Moonen for scanning the artwork; to my first editor, Anne Tucker, for her guidance and suggestions; and to Anna Comrie-Thomson for photos, including the four-seasons cherry trees.

I gratefully acknowledge the involvement of Mary Schumacher and Hospice New Zealand.

My patients, being the mirror of my soul, I thank for their extraordinary gifts.

Thank you, Wendy, for choosing me to accompany you on this journey. I love you.

With infinite gratitude to Sai Maa Lakshmi Devi. You teach me how to travel light.

INTRODUCTION

~ My own journey

I WAS FIVE YEARS OLD when I experienced my first deep loss.

It is 1942 and the Germans have occupied Holland. German Headquarters summon my father, who is a navy officer, together with many other high-ranked officers, to attend a weekend meeting in the south of Holland.

I walk with him to the tram shelter around the corner. "I'll see you tomorrow night," he says, giving me a kiss.

The meeting takes place in a train wagon with TRANSPORT printed on the outside and lasts for two days. His journey continues for the next three years in a concentration camp in Poland.

For weeks I go back to the tram shelter. Every night I pray to that unknown entity called God to do something, and tell myself that surely tomorrow he will be there. My father always keeps his promises.

It takes a long time, and a Red Cross letter, for me to accept defeat. I exchange hope and trust for anger and fear, and by now I very much doubt that the God my father so ardently believes in really exists.

My unexpressed anger and fear are fed by the many unpleasant things that happen during wartime, and are joined by a silent sadness. To keep my feelings under control I build walls around me, and through some cracks I cautiously survey my world.

I paint on a happy face for the outside world, having discovered that taking care of people, being nice and making them laugh is good medicine for them — and me.

In 1945 my father arrives home, looking like a scarecrow. He is riddled with fleas and bedbugs and cancer. The elimination of 'the crawly material' is easy but the cancer in both lungs and brain takes more then a simple pesticide. It is attacked by good surgeons with sharp knives, but being 1946 there is a lack of proper anesthetic drugs and no adequate analgesic medication, resulting in conditions which my father describes as "worse than the camp."

During these two years his faith in a loving and supportive God never falters, and even in his terrible agony I never once hear him complain.

Encouraged by the constancy of his belief, I start my prayers again in the hope that this time God will listen.

I am ten years old and I stand next to my father's hospital bed. A frame is being pulled up beside the bed to prevent him falling onto the floor. I'm watching my father moving around in his cage, my hands like claws around the iron bars.

I know he is going to leave me again, and this time there will be no tram shelter. And no promises. It is obvious that God has not been listening again and I am getting angry.

"God I need to talk to you and I want you to listen this time. Do you see my father, my father who loved you all his life, do you see how much pain he is in? And where are you? What are you doing? You are doing nothing, you can't even take his pain away. What kind of God are you? Well, I'm telling you now, I am going to do something. I am going to help people with cancer. That's my promise to my father."

Then I throw God away and forget my promise for quite some time.

But it does not forget me.

I become a doctor, determined to be a good and compassionate doctor. I love looking after people and I enjoy the feeling of being needed. I work very hard in Holland, for two years in the United States and eventually in New Zealand. My work starts to involve the care of terminally ill patients, in particular those with cancer and Aids.

My internal war continues behind the smiling exterior walls and I make sure I'm busy and don't spend too much time thinking about myself, or even worse, feeling the unresolved pain. At times it takes some effort to keep that rage inside, and consequently a low backache becomes my physical reminder that some rest could be appropriate. Often I feel embarrassed when my tears, using any opportunity to escape, trickle down my cheeks.

In 1985 my partner and I go to Egypt. I am fascinated by the Valley of the Kings, the tombs, the pyramids and the preparation for the ongoing journey of the soul.

Sailing down the Nile we meet a fellow passenger, an American woman from Boston. We talk about all sorts of things and when she learns I'm a doctor, she's very surprised that I haven't heard of Dr Elisabeth Kübler-Ross.

"She's a Swiss-born psychiatrist, famous for her work with the dying. She has written many books, leads workshops, and lectures all over the world. You must meet her."

I take another sip of my gin and tonic. "Yes," I answer casually, not giving it a lot of thought. "She sounds like a good person to meet."

Nine months later I happen to look in the paper and read an announcement: 'World-renowned psychiatrist, Dr Elisabeth Kübler-Ross visits Wellington'.

That evening in the Town Hall with 3000 people crammed in together, I'm eagerly waiting to hear what she has to say. With a noticeably Swiss accent, this small, dynamic woman speaks effortlessly for three hours about death and dying, about her work with the terminally ill and about the hardships and pain of daily living. She shares many stories with us and I feel moved by her total commitment to her work and her profound compassion for her patients. She sings the music of my soul.

Next year, 1987, I attend her five-day residential workshop, called 'Life, Death and Transition'. My ignorance leads me to assume I will learn a lot more about death and dying and consequently my patients will benefit from the experience.

Instead, I cry for five days. The walls are not smiling any more. Over the next fourteen years I have the great good fortune to train and work with Elisabeth and other members of her staff and become part of her team of facilitators.

During those first years of my training, Elisabeth and other facilitators create a safe place where I can cry and feel my pain, surrounding me with an unconditional love through which I can start to release my rage and fear. With Elisabeth's help I find my trust again — in humanity, in God and in myself.

Like Jericho, the walls come tumbling down and there is room for the light to enter and absorb the darkness. Light of knowledge, light of love and compassion, light of laughter and joy. My 'house' with a new foundation now has the sunlight streaming through the open windows, and the wind freely entering and playing in the previously locked-up rooms.

I become interested in different cultures and their rituals around death and dying. I study Eastern philosophies and spirituality and attend seminars and workshops around issues of grief and loss. My way of doctoring changes and I begin to place much more emphasis on 'being with and working in' the emotional and spiritual worlds of my patients.

But something is still missing.

I believe in the continuation of life, I believe in angels and the spirit world, I have a sense of consciousness and a sense of a loving presence. I have great respect and awe for this newfound deity, but even while I intellectually understand my own divinity, and full-heartedly accept the fact that God seems to be very approachable and present, God is still decidedly distant.

According to the mystics and saints, our search for God, for the experience of living in divine bliss, is the sole purpose of human life. So I keep searching: "Who and what is this energy we call God or Light or Allah or Yahweh? How and where can I find it? Who am I?"

In 1993 I am asked to talk about grief and loss with a group of nurses. Instead of the usual way of introducing themselves by name and specialty of work I take a different tack and suggest: "Take a few minutes to go inside and ask yourself why you really chose to become a nurse."

Many in the group are surprised by the answers and insights. Finally they look at me and a nurse in the front row says, "Your turn. Why did you become a doctor?"

A ten year old is waiting. I see her little claws around the bars of my father's bed. She turns to me and says, "I am going to do something. I am going to help people with cancer."

I know now that while I forgot that promise, that promise never forgot me. A soul decision, voiced by my ten-year-old self, has been patiently waiting for me to remember. I wonder if the answers I have been searching for, about who and what

God is, are also patiently waiting for me to remember. Waiting for me to be still and silent and listen.

It is said that the teacher always arrives when the student is ready. The day I meet meditation master Gurumayi Chidvilasananda, I know my search is over. Gurumayi is the spiritual head of Siddha Yoga, a path of discipline and study, of mastering the mind and senses with teachings and practices, of centering in one's heart.

As master and teacher, Gurumayi guides and teaches students to live in the awareness of the divinity both in themselves and others, enabling them to transform themselves and the world they live in.

I become her student and start my inner journey to the heart.

A journey to my authenticity, to joy, to freedom.

~ Communicating through art & poetry

WHY DO I WRITE ABOUT WENDY?

Is it the extraordinary wisdom she gained on her journey with cancer?

Is it her beautiful art, leading the way for readers to travel by?

Is it about hope and love, and Wendy choosing how to live and how to die?

Is it her strength and courage in accepting her cancer, but not allowing it to place any limitation on her living?

Or is it about what I learned from her?

This book is really a dance, a *pas de deux*, a duet.

The musical score, the different movements, I have written with gifts of wisdom I received from Gurumayi, Elisabeth and Wendy.

In every pause there is a breath of gratitude.

My hope is that this book will support anyone diagnosed with a life-threatening illness.

May it give hope to families where a child, grandchild, sibling or relative is diagnosed with cancer, or other life-threatening illness.

May it encourage health professionals, allowing creativity to enter the dialogue with their patients.

May it help us to hold onto hope, have faith in our own innate wisdom and let love be the key to every gateway.

First encounters

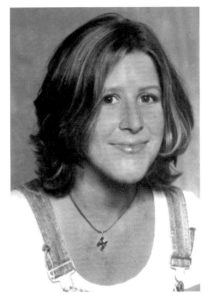

Wendy in 1991.

Studio 2005

MY PATIENT HAS JUST LEFT and through the open window of my studio I feel the soft early summer breeze. Birds are flying in and out of the little birdhouse which I filled with forgotten cake and an apple. Blackbirds are splashing around in the old ceramic birdbath.

I love my garden at this time of the year. The yellow and blue pansies, the orange calendulas, the red roses and sweet peas, the white daisies, and of course my pride and glory, the Japanese maples.

In 1995 I had the studio built in my garden for my counselling practice. It nestles in an abundance of colours, shapes and smells, and frequent visits from my winged and noisy friends.

A stained-glass butterfly which hangs against the window, reflecting sun and light, moves slowly in the wind. As always, it reminds me of Wendy. She loved to be here in this studio and insisted my golden retriever, Harvey, be present as well. This has been a place to share laughter, tears, silence and words.

I am aware how often I think of Wendy. How she travels with me through time, how past moments come alive again. Sometimes I think I hear her laughter.

It began in the winter of 1993.

August 1993

I have an appointment at my surgery with a new patient, a 16 year old who was diagnosed with cancer two years ago. Her name is Wendy Potter.

I read her medical history the hospital has sent me, and jot down some notes:

WENDY JOAN POTTER   D.O.B.: 7-7-77

Severe eczema and allergies since birth. Presently well controlled.

Asthma: Ventolin inhaler.

1991 July   Diagnosed with Hodgkin's disease after biopsy
             of gland in right groin. Investigation reveals
             bone marrow involvement.

      Aug   Chemotherapy started.

1992 Jan   Last treatment. No evidence of Hodgkin's disease.

      April Severe bout of shingles.

      Dec   Enlarged gland — left supra-clavicular area.

1993 Feb   Chest x-ray and CT scan: abnormal. Recurrence
             Hodgkin's disease. Start of chemotherapy.
             Wendy sees Mary Inglis, hospital counsellor.

      July   Biopsy of enlarged lymph nodes in right groin
             & left clavicle.

      Aug   Confirmed presence of Hodgkin's.

Suggested therapy:

1. High-dose chemotherapy with bone marrow transplant.

2. Total body nodal radiotherapy.

Family: Parents: Janet & Cyril Potter. Grandparents alive.
          Siblings: Lisa & Rachel — both older.

The last letter in the file mentions that after a long discussion, Wendy is still undecided about further chemotherapy; she feels unable to tolerate the stress and physical consequences associated with this treatment.

My work in both orthodox and complementary medical fields leads many patients to consult me when considering their treatment options.

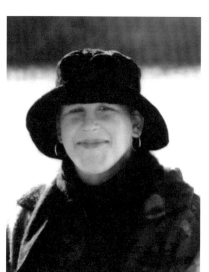

I get up from my chair and walk to the waiting room. It's lunchtime and there are only three people there. A man and a woman sit on either side of an attractive teenager.

She smiles at me, and I invite them all into my room. An extra chair is needed and my nurse brings a little wooden one which sits awkwardly between the two green upholstered chairs.

Wendy is a pretty, somewhat pale young woman wearing a dark blue, velvety hat which hides the loss of her hair. Clearly a price she has paid for her chemotherapy.

Her parents I estimate to be in their early forties. They look tired and strained. There is an unspoken sadness around them.

I can feel their apprehension: Another talk, another doctor. But … perhaps there is some hope?

I have questions about Wendy's medical history, her family background, her schooling. And during the next ten minutes all three create a picture of Wendy for me.

A teenager who, after two years of cancer, hospitals, chemotherapy and the disappointments of treatment failure, still loves life, still has hope, still can laugh. She spends a lot of time writing and drawing, and loves nature, music and lighthouses.

I turn to her. "When they did the biopsy in 1991, were you worried about the result? Did you ever think it could be cancer?"

"Oh, no, not at all. I thought it might be an infection or something. I think I went hysterical when the doctor called me and told me I had cancer. I was home alone and just screamed and screamed. Then I phoned Mum."

Janet looks at me. "I will never forget that phone call as long as I live."

Cyril adds, "I was numb with fear that this could happen to my daughter. Just total disbelief. Total shock."

Wendy talks about her treatment: her fear of the unknown and of hospitals.

It is the story of a carefree schoolgirl who lost her illusion of immortality, who lost her day-to-day contact with friends, and who knows that even if the cancer is not visible, she is different and will continue to be different from her peer group.

I glance at my notes. "In 1992, your cancer went into remission. Did things feel a little normal again?"

Janet answers. "There were always the dreaded hospital visits every two to three months, always reminding us that the cancer could come back at any time. I felt so relieved when everything was all right. Even though I tried to think everything was normal, it never really worked."

Wendy chips in, "I went back to school. I partied, drank, had boyfriends and tried to be the same as everybody else. That didn't work either."

Cyril shifts in his chair. "I so wanted to believe in the statistics. We were told the prospect of curing the disease was very high, in excess of eighty percent."

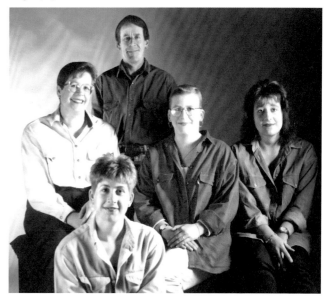

A family photo: Janet, Cyril, Wendy, Lisa, and Rachel in front, 1992.

We sit quietly, thinking of the sadness when a year later the cancer recurred and the 'normal' existence turned out to be an illusion.

"How did you cope with the side effects of your treatment?" I ask.

"I threw up after all my chemo treatments. Sometimes it was as soon as we left the hospital, before Mum or Dad could even get me in the car. I got injections for it sometimes, but they didn't work that well. Then my hair started to fall out."

The sadness and pain of the memory are visible.

"Every day there was more on my pillow, until one day I took a shower and afterwards all my hair was in the bath. I tried a wig but it wasn't me, so now it's hats."

"Well, you look good in them."

"Thanks. They're all right, but I'd prefer to have my hair back."

"Have you ever asked, 'Why? Why me?'"

Cyril's response is immediate. "I have. I've often asked why, why my daughter, why does it have to happen to our family? What have we done wrong?"

"Do you think you have done anything wrong?"

"No. No, I don't think that."

I turn to Wendy again. "Tell me what's happening for you now."

"I guess I'm still trying to get used to the words that are coming up now, like 'cancer' and 'death'. I know it's stupid, but I always thought that doctors knew all the answers and would just be able to fix what's wrong with me. It seems like I belong to the twenty percent of people for whom a cure might not be possible. I'm more scared of the treatment than I am of the cancer 'cause I hate hospitals and needles, and I feel sick just driving past the hospital. I've lost all faith in the treatment and I think I've lost faith in the doctors too."

I pick up the last hospital letter in her file and open it. "Have you thought more about your decision to accept or refuse further treatment?"

"Yes, I've thought a lot about it and I've talked with Mum and Dad. I'm sure the doctors are doing all they can and they're pushing me to keep going with the treatment, but I don't think I can continue. I want to understand cancer and find other ways to fight it. I stopped trusting my intuition and I need to start believing in myself again."

"Situations like this force us to find our wisdom, our voice, our truth. They force us to go within. Your creativity will help you, particularly your drawing and writing that you mention. I'd like to do some work with you involving your drawings."

"Like what?"

"Well, next time when I see you, bring some of your drawings. I might ask you some questions about what I perceive, what I see and what I feel from them. Perhaps there are some symbols or images I'd like to know more about. These questions and your answers will help you to journey within. It's a process from the conscious questions to the unconscious answers. I can't tell you how that process works, but I can tell you that it works. It's 'the language of the soul'."

Janet asks how long I've been working in this way with patients and their art, and I talk about my training and work with Dr Elisabeth Kübler-Ross, and how I met an American psychologist, Gregg Furth, about ten years ago.

Gregg taught me that drawings are a form of communication and that the language of the pictures is the language of our unconscious that speaks when the conscious voice fails. Carl Jung wrote about the realm of the unconscious and how it can be represented in art; according to him, images and symbols displayed in paintings, sculptures, poetry, dance, music, and many other forms are expressions that originate in our unconscious. He calls it 'the seat of creativity'.*

* Gregg M Furth *The Secret World of Drawings: Healing Through Art,* Sigo Press, Massachusetts, 1988.

Gregg also taught me that the expression of art is a valuable tool when we work with people faced with their mortality. It allows us to bypass the clever, conditioned mind which can take over and doesn't allow the emotions to speak. In a way it stops us from feeling the pain. And yet the often suppressed and hidden emotions need to come to the surface to clear the way to that inner place of wisdom and healing.

Wendy is clearly interested. "Okay, I'll bring my drawing book next time I see you."

"Good. I'm looking forward to seeing some of your creations."

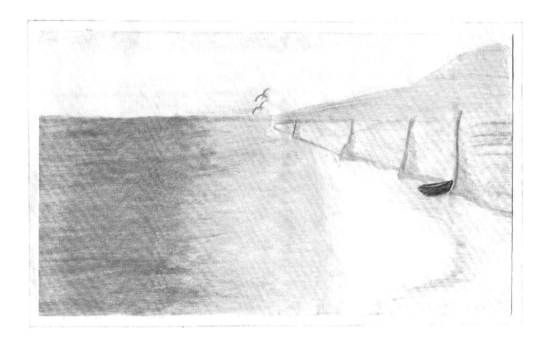

September 1993

A FEW WEEKS LATER Wendy returns wearing brightly coloured trousers, jacket and purple hat, her drawing book tucked under her arm.

I point at her hat. "Not bad."

"Eventually you'll see them all, unless my hair grows faster." She makes herself comfortable in one of the green armchairs.

"How do you spend your days?"

"I walk down the beach, go to the lighthouse, play piano and visit my grandparents, and I'm studying through the Correspondence School for a few hours a day."

"Do you miss your school friends?"

"Yes I do. I had fun at school, but I think my friends don't always know what to say or how to be with me … I look different and I guess I am different now." For a while she is lost in her thoughts.

"Can I see some of your drawings?"

The first one she shows me depicts a black boat on a beach.

"Tell me about the boat."

"It's stranded. No idea where it's going or how."

"What do you think that boat needs?"

"Oars and a rudder for direction, and maybe somebody to help push it into the sea."

"It might be quite easy when the tide is high."

"Yeah." She sounds a little surprised.

"Perhaps there is a piece of driftwood on the beach, which can be used as a rudder."

"Oh, so the choice is either be stuck on the beach or be out at sea with a piece of driftwood. Now that's attractive."

I don't answer.

Wendy points at the boat. "That's how I felt with the chemo, scared and stuck, and I don't want that any more. I'm ready to find that piece of driftwood."

She shows me two more drawings and in both, the light of the sun is reflected in the water. Rising or setting?

"What time of the day is it?"

"End of the day. The sun is going down."

"What else is going down?"

"My hopes, my dreams — like living in a lighthouse — things I wanted to do in life. I have to let them go. They're flying away like the birds in the drawing."

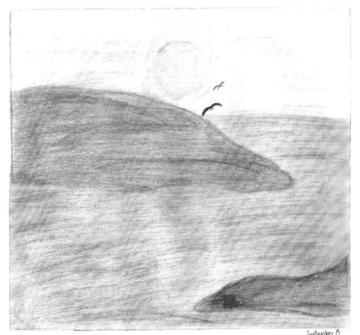

September 8
2. 34

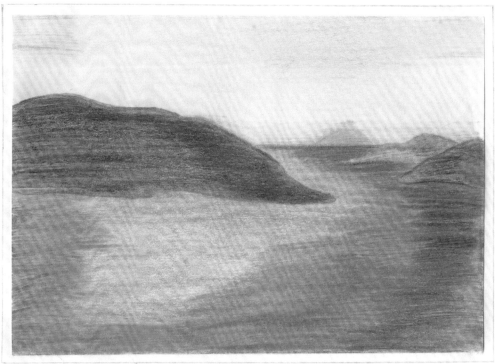

24 august 93

I put the second drawing in front of me. "The land is quite green."

"Yeah, well it might look healthy, but what's happening underneath?" She sounds cynical.

"And what's happening underneath?"

There is a sadness in her voice when she answers. "I don't know. I have good days when I feel almost normal, whatever 'normal' means when you have cancer. And then there are times I'm terrified and I can look at my body and have not the slightest idea what and where the cancer is. What the hell is it doing in my body? I hate not knowing what's going on. I have some lumps in my groin, perhaps that's a sign of more cancer, I don't know."

I get the sense that she is hoping that with one sweep of my medical wand I will provide clarity.

"I don't know what is going on in your body either, but let's talk about cancer in a different way. Cancer is a living energy and this living energy, these cancer cells, can invade your body. They create havoc and you get sick."

"What do you mean, 'invade'?"

"Imagine your body is a house with many rooms and doors and windows. You're having a party, and it's the party of living in good health and innocence. You're celebrating in your own unique way and having a good time, when cancer cells gatecrash your party. Unexpected and uninvited, they walk into your house and go from room to room, causing chaos. They enter your bedroom and you feel caught in the anguish of a nightmare you don't seem to be able to wake up from. They move to the kitchen and stop the food supply and you feel exhausted, down and depressed. They change the music and a cacophony of sharps, flats and minors stifle the song of your soul. They go to your living room and start reorganising your life. Remember, cancer cells are very alive and searching for a beautiful house where they want to live and settle for a while, which happens to be your body."

"This house isn't all that beautiful any more." Wendy points at her hat. "I've had better parties. So if the unwanted guests won't leave, what do I do now?"

"You need to meet this uninvited guest and find out who it is and what it wants. Remember, this visitor has moved in and decided to stay for a while. You, Wendy, are the owner of the house and you want to be in charge. Claim your house back. You need to decide where you want the cancer to live. Do you want it to live in the kitchen, in the bedroom, the living room, the music room? Or perhaps you have a room somewhere in the back of the house that you don't often use. Why not tell it to live there? Bed and breakfast in the back room!"

"Oh, no. I am not sharing my breakfast. I want to starve the cancer to death."

I laugh. "No, cancer cells are clever and they'll search for 'food' anywhere in your body, so why not give them what *you* want them to have? You'll have to find out for yourself what your cancer likes and doesn't like."

"What!?"

"Yes, that's right. You see, all cancers love negativity; they feed on hate and resentment and blame. So feed them laughter and feed them love. They despise the light, so switch on the lights in your house. Find your voice, find the song of your soul again."

"Well, I'm going to be busy, by the sound of it. And all that because I didn't close the windows."

She shows me a third drawing and smiles. "More green."

"Looks pretty healthy to me."

She studies her drawing for a while. "Yeah, and a good view from the top. With a bit of luck I might even see an old rudder lying around."

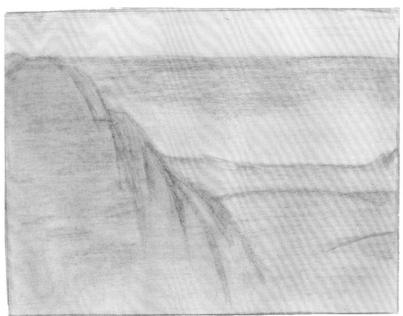

September 12
'Ngamu'

TRANQUIL

I gather smooth pebbles in the palm
of my hand
Cool continuous waves gently lap around
my naked ankles
Looking up
the cloudless sky is like
an enormous doorway
beckoning to be opened
Unharmed
I feel serenity
Untouched
I feel blessed
Unaware
I am isolated
The smooth pebbles I have gathered slowly
slip between my fingers into the water
                        one
                        by
                        One

1 July 1993

October 1993

"WELL, THAT WAS ANOTHER exciting visit to the hospital," Wendy announces, taking her coat off and throwing it over the back of her chair. "They couldn't have been any clearer: 'You will die fairly soon if you don't accept the treatment'."

"Do you believe the doctors?"

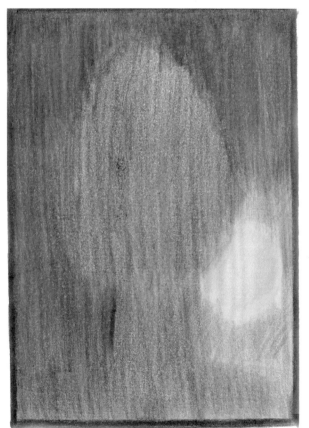

'Far Away'
5 October

She shrugs. "They've told me stuff before that turns out to be wrong, so why believe them now? The question is not if I believe them, the question is whether I trust myself to make the right decision."

"What does the word 'right' mean to you?" Wendy stares out of the window, where a pale watery sun is offering some warmth to the first buds on a small kowhai tree in the courtyard.

After a while she turns to me. "You talked about finding my music again and claiming back the song of my soul. That's what 'right' means. My intuition tells me not to go for more treatment, but my mind is not convinced yet, and of course I'm scared." She opens her drawing book. "That's me."

'Far Away' is written underneath the thickly accentuated frame.

"Where is the 'me' in the drawing?" I ask.

Wendy points at the tree, surprised.

"Why do you choose to be the tree when you can be the light?" She touches the paper, slowly feeling her way into a new identity. Finally she reaches into her bag, takes out her writing book and pushes it in front of me. "This is also about light and darkness."

To me, cancer is a stairway rising up into the unknown. The stairway could lead up to a sun shine filled room with arrangements of perfumed spring flowers everywhere. The air is fresh and outside the widening sky is of rich blue colouring. Birds glide with the ocean breeze and from this room you hear their busy chattering talk. The stairway could also easily lead to a darkened room in which there is no furniture. The air is sour and the floorboards unstable. There is one tiny window and when you look through the stained glass all you can see is a grey, concrete wall. You can sense crawling bugs in this room but never are able to see them. Twice I have ventured to the top stair believing I will be able to feel the warm, comforting sun shine on my skin but to my horror darkness has folded around me instead. At the moment I am sitting on the middle stair, halfway up and halfway down, undecided as to whether tor go up the stairway or descend down. I am still facing downwards...

20 August 1993

"Twice I believed the chemo would lead me upstairs to the sunshine. Do I trust myself enough to walk alone?"

I take a piece of paper from my desk and draw a large circle on the blank page in front of me. I divide it into four.

"Here's something that may help you. This is called a personality or four-quadrant model. Elisabeth Kübler-Ross used it for teaching purposes in her workshops. It's really about different ways we perceive and experience our world. The first one is the *physical* quadrant, our body, and how we observe and experience the world through our senses. We see, hear, smell, we taste and touch. The medical profession mostly focuses on this quadrant. It's only twenty-five percent of the whole of you."

Wendy leans forward on the desk, her head in her hands. "Imagine someone telling their lover, 'Sorry baby, only twenty-five percent tonight'."

I burst out in laughter. "Thanks, Wendy, you have added a whole new perspective to this model." I am still grinning when I point at the next quadrant.

"In the second quadrant, called the *emotional*, we feel and express ourselves through our emotions, like fear, love, grief and anger, among many others. This one here is the *intellectual*, where we try to make sense of the world through our logic. We ask questions, we rationalise, we analyse, we read books and we try to find the answers using our mind. And the last one is our *spiritual* quadrant. Here we experience the world through creativity, dreams, art and music, and through our connection with nature. We contemplate larger questions such as 'What is the purpose of my life? Is there a God? What is God? Who and what am I? Is there life after death?' The spiritual quadrant is a place for philosophy, values, intuition, wisdom and so on."

"And all this time I never knew I was so nicely squared up."

"It would be a lot easier if that were the case, but you, me, and most of humanity are not at all nicely squared up. There is a constant push and pull in there. There are the voices of your body, mind, heart and soul. All of them try to tell you how to be, what to do, and where to go. Then one day cancer enters the scene. You, more than anybody, know that disease doesn't only manifest itself in the physical sense. It creates an emotional chaos, the intellect goes overtime to find answers and solutions, and often we are so challenged in our faith that we wonder if God has completely forsaken us."

"Yep, that makes sense. I hate it. I hate feeling so useless and scared and frantic."

I point at the circle in front of her. "There is so much potential healing power in the spiritual quadrant. We can use nature, prayer, meditation, faith and our belief in God or in the universal energy. We can use the arts, music and our creativity. It's a place where we can surrender and ask for help, wisdom and guidance. I believe we are held and comforted and loved by something much bigger than ourselves. Our soul is not cared for by human hands."

Wendy is deep in her own thoughts. "I use nature to get to that place. I always feel better after I've been to the beach, and I think that's why I love four-wheel driving with Dad. We camp out, we sleep under the stars. A little roughing it must be good for my cancer." I reflect on my own love of nature, how in the early morning I adore the stillness of the dawn, and a little later the sound of the tui and bellbirds as they bring the surrounding bush to life.

Wendy points at the circle. "My mind tells me it's important to make a decision soon, and here —" she points at the emotional quadrant "— is a lot of dread and anxiety, and buckets of tears. Sometimes I'm so scared I feel numb."

I try to reassure her, explaining that deciding is a process in itself, which will take time. "It's like an apple falling off the tree; when it's ripe it will fall, and it doesn't need to fall a moment earlier. The answers will come when you are ready to hear them. Will you discuss your decision with your family?"

"Yeah, once I've thought about it more. They don't pressure me. I am the one who has to make that decision and I will." I slide the quadrant drawing into Wendy's folder.

"Do you have more drawings?"

"Yes, one more."

A bird's-eye view. It reminds me of the previous one where Wendy climbed the green hill.

"I had a wonderful dream. I was flying over the sea and the hills and everything was so peaceful. I knew I still had cancer but it wasn't a problem at all."

"Everything looks different from a distance, eh?" She nods. The boulders on the beach are enormous and block the exit. I wonder if Wendy will be strong enough to climb over them.

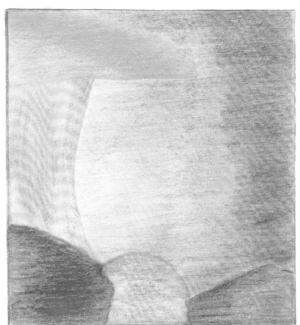

'I Believe In My Dreams
5 October '93

Along with regular visits to her naturopath, Wendy has been exploring alternative treatment options: Chinese medicine, diets, homeopathy. She is going inside her metaphorical house and switching all the lights on.

One day I have a message to call Wendy after surgery.

"Hi, how are you doing?"

"Not too bad. I wanted to tell you that Dad and I are going to the Hippocrates Health Centre, a clinic in Australia. It's known for it's complementary approach to cancer."

For the next ten minutes I'm given a rundown on the clinic's use of internal cleansing and detoxification, combined with special diets rich in mineral and vitamins. It involves fasting on juices then reintroducing raw salads and fruits.

All this combined with daily walking, swimming and steam baths.

I'm impressed. "Well, I hope you have a great time."

"I don't know about a great time. I'll just be doing what a girl needs to do to get rid of uninvited visitors."

The Hippocrates self-help and self-improvement programme focuses on nutritional, physical, mental and emotional balance and harmony. Their health centres are located in the USA and Melbourne, Australia.

Based on the belief that wholesome natural foods can restore and maintain health, all bread, meat, poultry, fish, dairy products, processed and cooked foods are excluded. Besides the cleansing and detoxification programmes, naturopathy, homeopathy, massage and spa-body treatments are available and recommended.

The seasons relate to the
stages of Wendy's journey,
not the calendar.

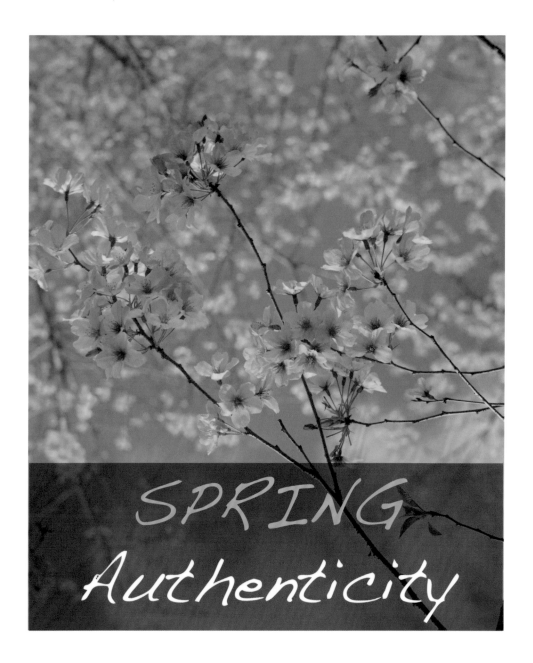

SPRING
Authenticity

December 1993

WENDY LOOKS VIBRANT when she bounces into my room. Her hair, which has grown back, is soft and shiny. When she turns her head, long silver earrings swing and touch the collar of her white linen shirt. Her sleeves are casually rolled up and velvety red burgundy pants complete the outfit. She glows with life.

She sits down and smiles at me. "Surprised? My Hippocrates diet isn't exactly French cuisine, but it works. I feel stronger every day, but poor Dad was also on the diet while we were there, and he lost so much weight. He's been living in the fridge since we got back. And I've decided not to have chemotherapy or any other hospital treatment at the moment."

"I'm glad you have come to a decision, Wendy. Did you talk it through with your family?"

"Not really. I told them my decision."

Wendy proceeds to tell me how she invited the family for a 'round the table' meeting. Candles were lit, tea was poured and Wendy informed her family about her decision. Although this announcement was made with great compassion for her family, it was obvious there was no room for negotiation, only discussion.

"I'm not sure if they all agree with my decision, but at least they can start doing something. Dad is busy reading the books he bought in the clinic and researching some different complementary therapies. And Mum has thrown herself into shopping and cooking all my special meals. She's happy when she can do things for me."

She leans back in her chair and absentmindedly plays with her left earring.

"So much is changing. I feel different and it's like there's a new me. A new owner living in my 'house'."

"Do you like the new owner?"

She gazes out of the window before she answers. "Yep. She trusts herself again. The world isn't as scary any more. She accepts that things have changed and that makes her sad, but she is determined to make the best of what there is. And she has taken over the kitchen again."

Wendy pulls her green drawing book from her bag and opens it in front of me. "I have lots of drawings for you."

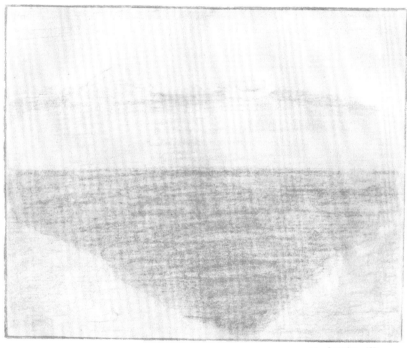

Water, as in a chalice, held by land ... overflowing on both sides.

"It must be hard always to be so careful. Careful about what you eat and don't eat, and careful to get enough rest." She nods. There are tears in her eyes and I give her some tissues.

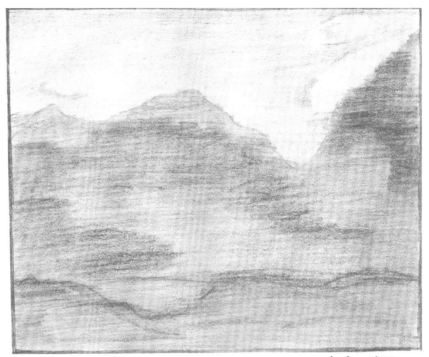

1 december

"It's okay to cry. Tears have to flow, like water. Then you have some more space inside."

She smiles weakly. "And then I get mad and I fill that space with anger. Like that." She points at her second picture.

"I just want to be normal and go to school and parties. Get drunk, smoke, have late nights, do stupid things. But when I do meet my friends, it's not the same and it makes me sad. I've changed."

"Yes, you have." I turn the page. "Where are you in this picture?"

"Here," she points at the brown earth near the bottom of the drawing.

For quite some time Wendy stares at it. "I wonder if the grass is greener on the other side."

"Is it?"

"No, I'm happy where I am. It's where I've decided to be." She turns the page and points to her next drawing with a beautiful orange sky.

"This is my favourite time of the day. I feel at peace when I watch the sunset."

"The hills are very beautiful in that light."

She smiles. "The light is holding the hills, protecting them.

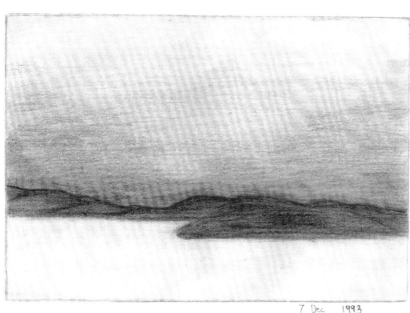

7 Dec 1993

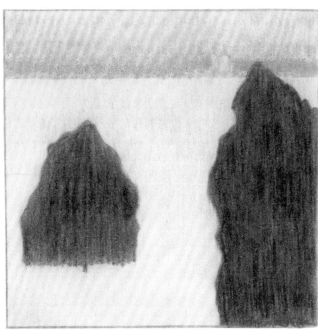

12 Dec' 93

"This is the last one, I did it a few days ago."

I study the picture. "Is that little rock connected with the land?"

"No. It stands by itself."

"It must be quite strong. There could be some undercurrents."

"Uh huh, and high waves too. The other rock is not too far away. Just like my mum."

I examine Wendy before she leaves. There's no sign of active disease.

"Are the glands still there?"

"Yes, you have one in your groin and one in your neck. They've been there for a while but haven't changed, so that's a good sign. I'd like you to go to the laboratory though, just for a routine blood test. Last one this year."

March 1994

"HI, SORRY FOR THE WAIT. I'm running late today."

She puts her bag down. "No worries, I have time."

"I've been thinking about you and I'd like to tell you one of my stories. It's not about a house this time. This one is about a bus."

"I hope it's running on time." She pulls her legs underneath her in the chair and settles back.

I chuckle. "Get on that bus Wendy, and enjoy the ride.

"You know, when we talk about ourselves we use the word 'I,' as in 'I, Wendy; I, Hetty'. But in some ways, the 'I' is really a 'we'. 'We, Wendy; we, Hetty'. There are many 'Wendys' inside you, like a bus full of people. All these passengers are really parts of us, parts of you. There's an angry one, there's a happy one, a sad one and a content one. There's a peaceful one, a scared one, the judge, the blamer, the clown and the martyr. There's the one who laughs, the one who cries, the wise one, the courageous one, the one who's forgiving and the one who holds resentment. And there's the one who loves, who cares. There's a shy one, a compassionate one, a silent one and a talker, and many more. Each of them sees and perceives the world around her in different ways. As the saying goes: 'the world is as you see it'. Therefore each of these passengers will respond, react, and express herself according to how she experiences the world. So how you feel depends on who's driving your bus."

"Makes sense to me."

"But you are in charge of all those passengers and you can change the driver whenever you want. You're ultimately the observer of all that's happening. You observe all the passengers, their conversations, their ups and downs, their wants and needs and likes and dislikes of each other and the world. So, if you don't like how you feel and want to change, change the driver. There's one rule — you can't throw anybody off the bus. Sometimes you might think you can get rid of them by pushing them out the front door, but they always enter again through the back door. However, you can tell them to sit in the back of the bus and be quiet. Often we can get so involved in the ride that we completely forget to change the driver. Or there are times you don't want to change the driver. It's important to respect the sad and the scared ones and let them drive as well. They need to show you how they see the world."

Wendy grins. "Well that's a relief. Now I know it's okay to be full of myself."

She opens her drawing book. "Quite a few different drivers that day."

"At this point in your life, it's almost 'normal' to go up and down. Not particularly pleasant, but almost to be expected. It's never a straight line anyway, more like a wave, which hopefully will flatten out more."

"Until the next tsunami."

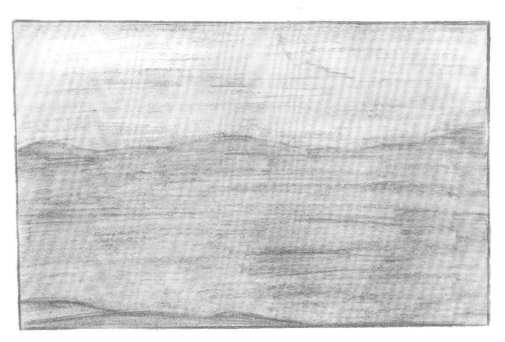

31 January 1994

She turns the page to a drawing of a lighthouse and I remember her dream of living in one.

"Why do you want to live in a lighthouse?"

"It's very safe inside, and light and warm, and the sea is crashing around it but nothing bad can happen. It's strong."

"Where are these birds going?"

"This one's flying towards the land. It's going home for a while."

For some time Wendy contemplates the birds and the lighthouse. "But the other one stays with the light."

I wonder if this picture might represent her search for identity, a longing to know 'who am I?' There's an awareness of an inner and outer reality, an inner and outer Wendy. The outer Wendy flies back to the land. This is the Wendy who will drive her bus. The other Wendy starts the journey inside, the journey to find truth, the journey to find the light.

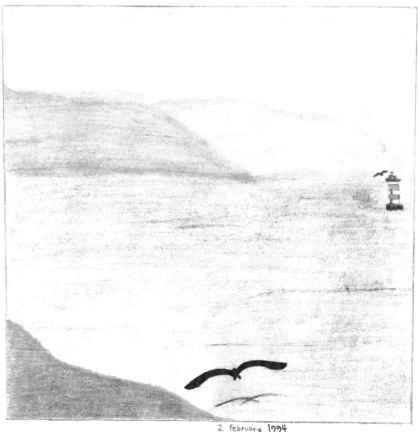

2 February 1994

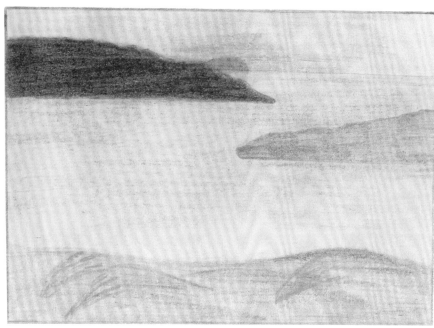

7 february '94

"I did one more, and some writing as well."

She puts the open book in front of me. "Does it have a story?"

Wendy points at the brown earth at the bottom of the drawing. "That's where I'm standing, watching the sun go down. I feel my feet again, touching the earth."

"Do you feel more in charge of your life now?"

"Yes. After chemo I felt so disconnected from everything, but I feel more secure now. I'm reading and exploring different philosophies, religions, and belief systems. Can I read you one of Buddha's teachings? I found it the other day:

> What we are today, comes from our thoughts of yesterday,
> Our present thoughts build our life of tomorrow.
> Our life is the creation of our mind.

"Isn't it amazing?"

"Well, the ancient sages teach us the mind with all its thoughts, ideas, concepts and beliefs can be our friend or our enemy. Every moment in our lives we have the choice of which one we engage with. Do we view the world through the eyes of the heart? With kindness, love and generosity? Or do we view it through eyes filled with anger, fear, resentment and negativity?"

"Yeah, I'm starting to really get that, but it's hard to put it into practice and live it."

"I agree. Some people say it takes many lifetimes."

"Cancer certainly helps you go faster. I don't know if I'll have a lifetime." She returns to her notebook. "I like this one too. I'm not sure who wrote it, but I think it might have been Voltaire:

> Each player must accept the cards life deals him.
> But once they are in the hand, he alone must decide
> how to play the cards in order to win the game.

"I have faith in my cards, Hetty."

I feel moved by her sincerity. Or is it her innocence?

"And I have faith in you, Wendy."

It starts to rain, and for a moment we both watch the drops fall on the leaves of the rhododendrons outside.

I close Wendy's file. "I believe it's very important to have faith. It connects us with our innate inner wisdom. I'll give you one of my favourite sayings to take home, from Rabindranath Tagore, an Indian writer. He said: 'Faith is the bird that feels the light when the dawn is still dark'."

There's a sudden lightness around her and her laughter fills the room. "There's my bird again."

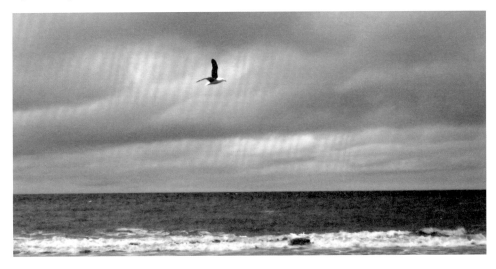

Studio 2005

A GENTLE RAIN IS FALLING and the sky is grey. I listen to the staccato of the drops on the roof of my studio. The sun, given a small window of opportunity, shines through occasionally. I watch the birds flutter around a 'fatball,' a concoction made up by the butcher, which hangs on a small iron hook on the almost leafless elm. There's a definite hierarchy: blackbirds and starlings seem to have the monopoly above the sparrows and finches who wait patiently in the outer circles. They clearly have faith that the bigger birds will depart and give them their chance for breakfast. Wendy loved to watch the many-coloured finches fluttering around the birdbath and the surrounding trees. I sit down and reacquaint myself with her 1994 hospital reports and letters.

May 1994

WENDY AND I HAVE started meeting in my lunch hour. It gives me more time to spend with her, and to enjoy the freshly baked scone or muffin she invariably brings. "Feels like ages ago since I saw you last." Wendy declares, pushing her chair closer to my desk. "I've been busy."

"Tell me. And by the way, this is divine." I savour a still-warm raspberry muffin.

"I know, I've had two already. Well, I'm starting to enjoy life again. Still doing lots of things with my sister, Lisa, but I'm going out more in the evenings with a guy called Reuben. He's an artist studying graphic design."

"When did you meet him?"

"Two years ago. I was in remission after the first series of chemo. He's wonderful and always there for me. When I'm sad or tired, he'll come and cheer me up. He sends me lots of funny letters and clever cartoons and it doesn't make any difference to him that I have cancer. I guess he loves me just the way I am. I've been to the hospital as well. Did they send you a letter?"

"Yes, they did. Here it is: 'Clinical examination shows no evidence of disease progression.' That's a good report."

"Yep. Considering the commotion I caused by refusing treatment. Oh, can you do a prescription for my inhalers, I forgot to ask the specialist."

"Sure." I reach for my prescription pad and write it out. "How is your asthma?"

"Really good. I use the blue one only as needed." She grabs her yellow backpack and takes her books out. "Some work for you, Hetty. I did quite a few drawings."

"Show me." I put my elbows on the desk, chin in my hands.

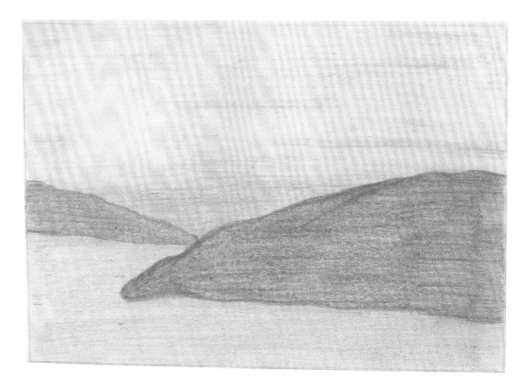

The sun is higher in the sky than in most of her previous drawings. There is more balance in the composition.

"I felt really good drawing this. I was at peace with everything."

"Do you often feel that way?"

She ponders my question. "I feel at peace when I don't think too much, when I don't try to get it right all the time." She laughs. "Maybe I just need to stop thinking. Can you give me a prescription?"

"Medical school doesn't teach doctors to write that sort of prescription. As a matter of fact the emphasis was on thinking, not feeling."

"So when did you change back to feeling?"

"When I met Elisabeth Kübler-Ross. She helped me — forced me, I should add — to finally examine my life and the pain and anger I held inside. And now my patients help me to remain in my heart."

Wendy is listening intently. "Perhaps that's what it's all about, to find your heart and stay there."

"Hmm, sounds a good place to call home."

"I did this one in watercolour, it was fun. I like it."

A big sun reflects its light onto the water. Although it's within a frame, some of the water spills over the borders. An early sign of Wendy starting to free herself from restrictions and widening her view of the world again?

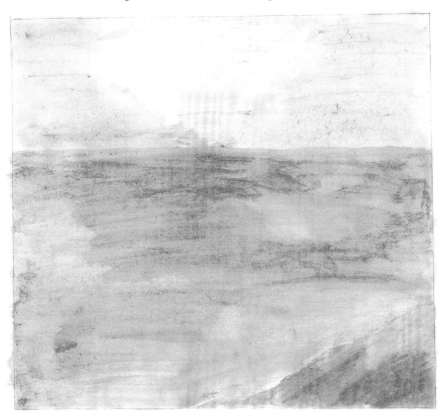

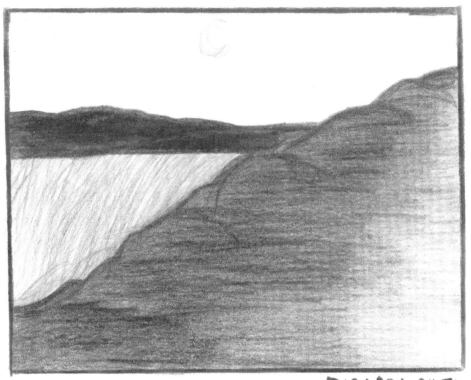

I9 APRIL 94

She turns the pages. "Those two are the latest."

"At what time did you draw those?"

"Oh, that one at dawn and the other later in the evening. See '10.24,' it's written underneath. I did it with candlelight. I've stayed up quite a few nights over the last month or so."

I give her a curious look and Wendy reveals her need to observe the starlit sky and ever-changing moon. She views the awakening of the dawn, the first hesitant rays of the early sun, the beginning of a whole new day. "I'm exploring another world and every night is different. I feel connected to something vast. Like infinity, always expanding. Difficult to find words for it."

I pull her drawing book a little closer to me. Both drawings are thickly framed. Safety seems important while exploring new worlds. "These clear patches in the sky are quite remarkable. As you said it is 10.24pm, it must be dark." For a long time she is still, communicating with her drawing.

It feels like a dialogue in silence. Finally she turns away and says, "I need to go deep into that darkness to feel the light." There is a stillness in her.

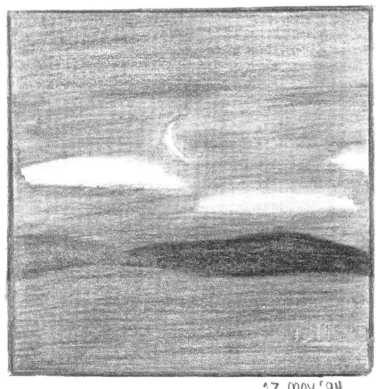

17 MAY '94
10·24

This is an important stage in the course of an illness. When faced with their mortality, patients often start to explore their mystical, hidden and spiritual dimensions. A journey from the light to the dark and from the outer to the inner world. A longing for truth, to know that which is beyond the known and to experience that which is beyond the senses.

Questions like: *Who am I? What is the purpose of my life? Is there a God? Is there life after death?* are frequently the incentive for this quest.

Before Wendy leaves she asks: "I want to know more about complementary ways of healing. Do you know anyone who works with crystals or gemstones?"

"Yes, Raven, she's a good friend of mine."

Raven is a gifted healer, even though she maintains her main purpose in this life is to be a mother. "She's very knowledgeable in the use of crystals, gemstones, meditation techniques and creative visualisation."

Wendy is pleased. "Just the person I want to meet. She might teach me to travel to new and exotic dimensions."

I have a strange feeling that that's just what Raven will do.

Gemstones act as a lens through which colour and light can be channeled. When used in conjunction with visualisation and breathing techniques, they are powerful tools for our physical and emotional aspects. Initially this will be the main focus with Wendy, to endeavour to strengthen her immune system. Later Raven will concentrate on meditation/journeying techniques to help Wendy expand her awareness and move beyond this dimension.

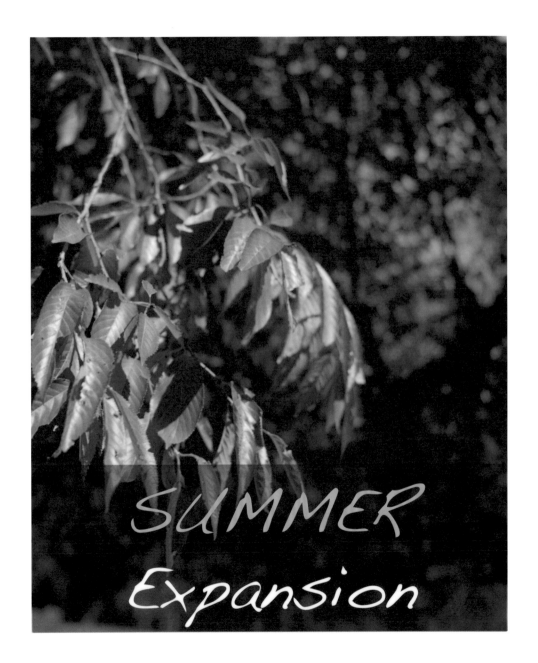

SUMMER
Expansion

August 1994

"KEEPING YOURSELF BUSY?"

Wendy draws up a chair. "Yes, you'll be pleased to hear I walk at least an hour every day. I'm studying for my School C in November and, because I'm such a good girl, I treat myself to some chocolate and watch television."

"I'm glad you've got your priorities sorted out!"

Wendy gives me a benevolent smile and continues. "I've done quite a lot of four-wheel driving with Dad. I have moments in the bush when I don't feel like a person who's got cancer."

"What do you mean?"

She looks out the window. Raindrops are slowly running down the glass. "It's like the rain outside. I'm watching it and yet at the same time I feel sort of detached. I talked about it with Raven. By the way, I really like her. We meditate together and I learn to work with my 'magic rocks'; that's what Lisa calls my gemstones. Raven gave me a book to read, *Moments of Truth*.* It makes me think a lot about time and life and death."

I lean back in my chair, holding her gaze. She's quiet for a while. "I know now if I get sick again and face death, it's only my body that will die. And although I don't know how and where, I know that I will continue like the nymph husks left behind when the cicadas fly to freedom."

"You've a good eye for what nature teaches us. Do you have someone to talk about these things with?"

"There's always Lisa, but she's planning to go overseas. I'll really miss her, but she needs to go. She's stayed in New Zealand for me."

I take a letter from the hospital out of her file. "Wendy, I received this from Oncology. At your last check-up it was noticed that the glands in your right groin are getting larger. This could mean a recurrence of your Hodgkin's disease."

*Excerpts from *The Rubaiyat of Omar Khayyam,* explained by Paramahansa Yogananda.

"Yes, they told me."

"Are you scared?"

"No, I'm not particularly worried. I feel better in myself all the time, less tired, becoming stronger. I absolutely do not want any more investigations."

"You'll still have to go for check-ups."

"I know, and I'm always nervous. The hospital's still an awful place. It reminds me of my treatments and injections, and that horrible feeling of being so dependent."

"Your body remembers. Cells have their own memory."

"I wish my cells had something more cheerful to remember."

She opens her drawing book. She's written the words: 'TO LIVE FOR' underneath the latest drawing.

"What a spectacular sky! What time of the day is it?"

"It could be the beginning or at the end of the day. Does it really make a difference?"

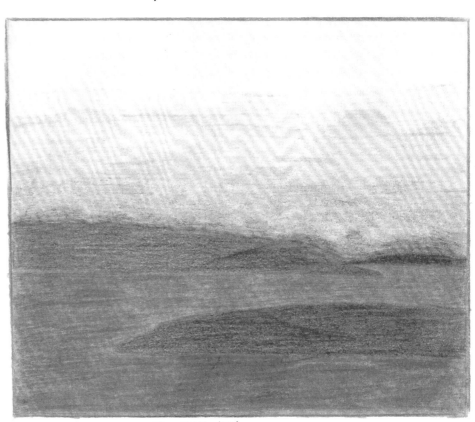

10 JULY 1994
'TO LIVE FOR'

Studio 2005

To HELP ME WEAVE Wendy's tapestry, her mother Janet has given me all of Wendy's writing — her diaries, poems, stories and her drawing book. Reading my notes and going through her drawings, I find the one she did on 8 November 1994, with its sun bright and full in the left-hand corner.

Elisabeth Kübler-Ross frequently used art and drawings in her work. She observed that when the patient starts to draw the sun in the top left-hand corner, a lasting transformation has often taken place and there's no longer a deep fear of death; the 'great unknown'. My own experience with patients has taught me that almost without exception there will still be the fear of being labelled and treated differently as 'the one with cancer'. There will be fear of possible changes in relationships with life, family, and friends. And there's always the fear of pain and the progression of the illness.

Thinking back, Wendy's only strong fears were those of hospitals and treatments, of losing control of her life, and of not being able to make her own decisions. The 'unknown' was still unknown, but she had no fear of it. From late 1994 onwards this became more obvious in her writing and drawings. Her insights, our talks and her writing all revealed a maturity far beyond her age.

Lisa told me once: "Wendy was not your typical teenager. Yes, she yearned for and thought about friends, fun, parties, someone to fall in love with. At the same time she was very strong, very wise and very spiritual."

December 1994

MY NURSE INFORMS ME that Wendy called and asked to see me today. "She wants you to check her glands. I think she said she's going away for a few days. I put her at the end of your list."

"I felt these glands in my neck, not sure how long they have been there. Can you have a look?" When I examine her there are indeed several slightly enlarged glands on both sides of her neck, as well as the previously found gland in her groin. I tell her that this most probably means a recurrence of her cancer. I see the fear, sadness and disappointment in her face. The fragile hope that it may have been a virus has been squashed.

"Hetty, I don't want any more treatment. I know that I made the right decision a year ago not to have any more chemo. I'm not changing my mind now. I can only speak for myself, but I don't have any faith or trust in that form of treatment. I felt it almost killed my body, my mind and my soul."

I hear her determination and know this 17 year old has made up her mind. After a moment she continues: "These glands mean the cancer is perhaps more active again, but I'm getting stronger and my body feels healthy. I can do 'normal' things again, like walking for hours, going out in the evenings and not being exhausted. My diet, exercises, meditation, writing and drawing are all helping me. And I've decided to go back to school. It'll give me more structure and focus in my life and it'll be fun to see my friends again. I feel almost normal, to be able to go back to school again." She pauses and catches my eye. "Almost," she repeats softly.

She's quiet for a while. "I'm happy at home, there's so much love. It works for me. My family helps me to feel whole again."

"I know that. Love is still the key and master player in the game called 'living.' I'd like to suggest that over the holidays you talk with your family again and contemplate your decision."

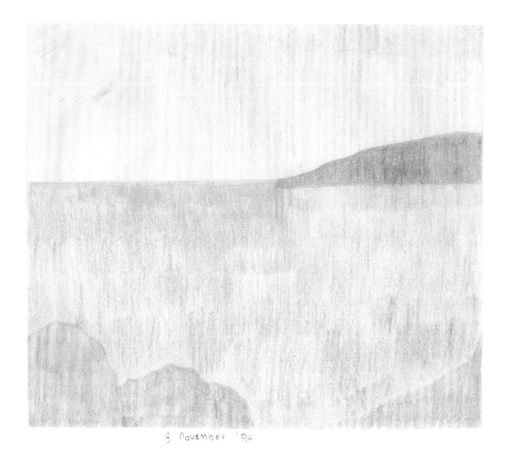

9 November '94

She shows me her latest art. Her drawing with a sun in the left-hand corner confirms my feelings about the changes happening in her. There's lightness, with less emphasis than usual on the land or water.

"How do you get off the beach?"

"I have to climb over those boulders," she answers. "The sun's warming them. It'll be easy." She winks. "I might just walk on the water; it's been done before."

"I called this one 'nightlove'. I've been looking at the moon again. It's a guardian in the night, silently watching me. Sometimes my cancer feels as far away."

She turns the page. "And this one's the early dawn, the sun is rising."

"Will it be a good day, Wendy?"

"Yeah. Look, there's so much light in the dawn, it awakens the land. The creation of a whole new day."

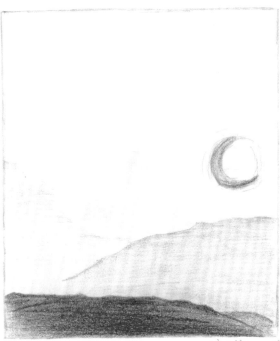

6 December   nightlove ♡

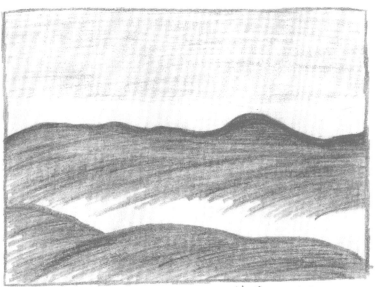

Akatarawas
27 December '94

A few weeks later I receive a letter from the Oncology Clinic, confirming my findings of that day:

11 December 1994

Wendy has a node in the right inguinal region, and also bilateral cervical nodes. I am afraid this is highly suggestive of relapsed Hodgkin's disease, especially as the node in the right inguinal region has increased in size over the past three months. Wendy is quite adamant that she would not consider further chemotherapy.

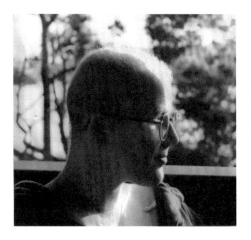

"They had told me that I would lose all my hair, but they can't tell you how it feels when you look in the mirror."

February 1995

I'M RELIEVED TO SEE THAT Wendy has asked Janet to come along with her today. I want to discuss treatment again and wonder how the family feels about the decisions Wendy has made.

"I got the letter from the Oncology Clinic. Your cancer has almost certainly relapsed. I'm so sorry about that. Last time we talked about treatment. Have you given it a little more thought and discussed it with your family?"

Both Wendy and Janet nod.

"Yes, I've done all that, and my decision to refuse treatment hasn't changed. You have all my medical notes and letters there …" she points at her file "… but I've a different story to tell. The endless blood tests, the bone marrow, all those scans. And then the biopsies, and twice the wounds got infected. I can't tell you how scared I was every time I walked into that hospital. I kept telling myself 'Just get through this, everything will be okay, you'll be home in a few hours.' The side effects of the chemo, I don't think I ever vomited so much in my life, nor have I ever been so bloody tired. And then my hair started to fall out. They had told me that I would lose all my hair, but they can't tell you how it feels when you look in the mirror. But I really believed that everything I went through was worth it and that the chemo was working."

Janet and I are both listening. She has tears in her eyes as Wendy speaks. "I just don't believe in orthodox medicine any more. I know the doctors want to help, but I don't want it. I accept the possible consequences that they repeatedly spell out to me, and I want to have control of my life and make my own choices about how I treat my body."

We sit there for a moment, Wendy's words resounding in the silence. I turn to Janet. "It must be hard for you and the rest of the family."

"Last year was almost a 'normal' year. Lisa left for her trip and Rachel left to live with her boyfriend. Cyril and I weren't always watching Wendy and worrying about her. I think we all relaxed a little, apart from the hospital visits every three months. I remember the relief when there was no sign of any recurrence of the cancer. We almost believed that life could become normal. Now it's all unknown again." Her anguish is palpable.

"Yes. The not-knowing is the hardest part. Do you support Wendy's decision not to have any more treatment?"

"Oh yes, whatever decision she makes, we'll support her. We've talked about everything, but Wendy has always made her own decisions in her own way, in her own time. Cancer's not changing that." They laugh.

Wendy's laugh fades. "I'm sure a lot of people of my age would decide differently. That's their choice and I respect that, but I need a good quality of life, which I know

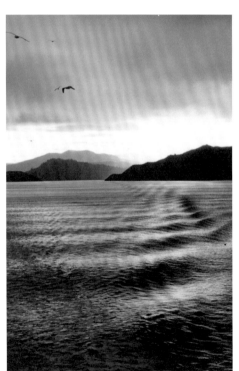

I can create for myself. And I believe in all the other complementary ways that I 'work' with my cancer, which includes coming to see you. I know how I want to live my life, as short as that might be. At the same time I get scared when they tell me what will happen if I don't accept the treatment."

"I believe most of us would feel like that. Remember your drawing of the two birds?"

"I do. With the lighthouse."

"In your drawing, one bird stayed with the lighthouse, close to the light, and the other returned to the land. The one in the light has the innate wisdom of the soul. It knows. The other bird needs to live on the land and participate in all its dramas and adventures. There is laughter and there are tears. There are many obstacles, and yet that bird will fly high. It will feel fear and dance with joy. It will experience the eternal cycle of seasons, the spring of hope, the summer of abundance, the autumn of letting go and the winter of stillness. I believe your life will be a balancing act between those two birds."

She stares at me, listening intently. "And ultimately they will be reunited."

April 1995

TODAY WHEN I EXAMINE Wendy I notice a few more small lumps on both sides of her neck. She has a dry, irritable cough. Her chest is clear on examination. "It doesn't sound too bad, but we'd better get a chest x-ray." I wonder what's going on in her life, as she appears more drained than when I last saw her. "Is school more difficult than you expected?"

"A little." She tells me about how she's getting involved again in school life and about the challenges she's confronted with. She's going out more. She drinks, goes to some parties and has late nights. She starts to feel tired and tries to pull back a little, but there's persistent peer pressure to keep up this lifestyle. Apart from the physical limitations she's experiencing, there's a much more painful awakening. "It's not the same any more. Lots of things have changed for me. I'm not always interested in parties, getting drunk or smoking pot. I feel old when I'm with my classmates and friends. I don't belong there any more."

"Do you feel lonely?"

"Not really, I've been asking myself that same question. I've accepted that school life is finished. It does make me feel more alone."

She hands me her journal. "I wrote this down the other day. It made me cry."

I read the poem, and the stillness lingers after she has closed her journal. I take the top sheet out of her opened file. "I see you've been to the hospital again. I understand your specialist explained the risk that you could develop quite extensive disease by refusing more treatment. That must have been a difficult visit for you."

"I'm angry because of the way they talked to me in the hospital. I know they mean well, but I'm mad."

MASK
The mans face smiles
with laughter
He admires the sky
earth and ocean
He walks with pride
and dignity
His mind is complete
with understanding
Every one thinks he is
happy
But deep down inside the
man is dead
The man always feels
alone

"What else do you feel angry about?"

"I'm angry that I have cancer and that I can't live my life the way I want to. And I'm scared of what might happen. I guess I'm scared of not knowing when things might happen."

"Are you scared of dying?"

"No, not really. I think living is scary and much more difficult."

We both look out the window where rain is creating puddles on the path outside. Two college girls are walking back to school. They're laughing, talking loudly, unmindful of their mortality. And yet death, like a shadow, will always be right behind them.

Wendy continues, "I don't want to feel angry because I have cancer. I don't want to be envious of other people's lives." I lean forward over my desk and touch her hand.

"Remember your bus? It's full of different Wendys. Some of the angry, sad or envious ones need to drive for a while."

"But sometimes it doesn't even feel like the real me who feels all this. Who is the real me anyway? Who am I?"

"These are probably the most important questions we can ever ask. It's been written in centuries-old scriptures and taught by many wise beings that these questions hold the answers to the purpose of our birth and to the purpose of life itself.

"I think I've told you that I facilitate five-day workshops organised by Elisabeth Kübler-Ross, and during those days we give quite a few talks and teachings on different subjects, among others, about our emotions. I made this teaching into a story. Easier to remember. It's really a story about God and a suitcase. Want to hear?"

"Yes," she says, leaning back in her chair, and I begin.

> There's a beautiful place, where we, Beings of Light, live. Some call this place heaven and others call it paradise.
>
> One day we decide to go back to planet Earth to do some more learning. Earth is where the school is. We go to some of the angels and say, "I'd quite like to go back for a while."

"Sure. What would you like to learn this time?"

"Well, in this coming lifetime I want to learn 'such and such' and I want to experience 'this and that'."

Together with these angels we write a soul script and we prepare ourselves for departure to Earth. When the time comes to leave, we walk to the gate and God is there. God speaks: "My child, where are you going today?"

"Good morning, God. I've decided to go back to Earth for a while. I've discussed it with the angels. Here is my script."

God regards this. "Yes, yes, it's a good script, not an easy one. I'd like to give you a present. Something to help you live your script. I'll give you a little suitcase." You're terribly excited. God opens the suitcase. "I'll show you what's in it. These are some tools you can use on planet Earth. They are called anger, fear and sadness. There are also a few tools you can use when you're very jealous and envious of other people. The whole suitcase is wrapped in love; it is called Love. You can take this with you to Earth and at the right time, at the right moment, you can use one of those tools to help you to express how and what you feel. There are screams for when you are scared and tears for sadness, loud noises for anger, and lots of smiles and laughter for when you feel happy and safe. After you've used your tools, pop them back in the suitcase, ready for the next time. See, I've written your name on it, same name as on your script. The script and the suitcase go together and are especially for you."

"Thank you very much, God. I promise I'll use it a lot. Well, I've got to go now but I'll see you when I come back."

And just when you start to walk through the gate, we hear God say: "Haven't you forgotten something?"

You're surprised. "Did I forget something, God?"

"You forgot to give me your memory, which contains everything about you: who you are, what you are, the purpose and meaning of your next life and who and what I am. Going back to Earth is like going back to school. You're there to learn. But if you know all the time who you really are and who and where God really is, then there's nothing to learn. And that is really all that you need to learn on Earth anyway. So it's more like a game where you, with the help of your script and your suitcase, try to remember the answers to: *Who am I? Who is God? What is the purpose of my life? Who is the real me?* Of course, when you're finished with your work on Earth and you arrive back here I'll give you your memory back. But I hope you'll remember some, or even all of this, while you're playing on Earth."

Wendy laughs. "I like this story."

"Good!"

So, you give your memory to God and while you're stepping through the gate, you hear God's last words:

"Blessings and good luck my child, and remember I love you. You will never be alone. I am always with you. My love is the beating of your heart. I am in all forms and I am in the formless. I am the tears of sorrow, the laughter of a child, the sound of war and the song of freedom. I am your silence. I am in all people. Meet me in their eyes. I will tell you a secret: all the answers are inside you."

You feel very safe. You know you'll never be alone and you think: 'I must remember that all the answers are inside me.' And so you arrive in the family you've chosen to incarnate in, suitcase and all. It's the start of your journey, the first page of your script. It'll very much depend on this family and other caregivers and guardians we're involved with, as to how and when we use our little suitcase. If we enter into a family where there's a lot of love, we might just glance at the suitcase. We might not even have to open it. However, if we enter a family with a lot of anger and we get frightened, we might need every tool in the case.

Most of us, when we innocently open our little suitcase to use our tools, are in for a big surprise. It's very obvious the big people don't want us to use any tools at all. They tell us if and when we're allowed to open our suitcase. They tell us which tools to use and for how long, and sometimes we're not allowed to have a suitcase at all. We get terribly confused and our suitcases get very messy.

Most people we meet have forgotten how to use their tools in the right way, at the right time, at the right place and in the right amount. Actually what's happened is that people have started using their tools to control and hurt others; to create fear and hate, and they forget that the name of the suitcase is Love. Over time most of us forget to look within for answers. Unaware of who we really are, we live the dream or experience the nightmare. So few of us have stayed awake. How do we wake up?"

Wendy interrupts, "Cancer wakes you up."

"Cancer does wake us up. We most often wake up because of a crisis. It can be death, illness or loss. It can be a natural disaster or war, and then we remember to care, love and trust again. I believe that you chose a family where you are allowed to express yourself and use all the tools you have. Open your suitcase and be angry. Shout; walk along the beach; scream in the wind; talk to people you trust. Anger that stays in the body gets terribly mixed up. It can become rage or depression. You don't want that to happen.

When you feel sad, use the endless supply of tears. And when you feel lost, when everything becomes too much and you feel worried and scared, talk to the moon, talk to the stars, listen to the wind and feel the rain. Touch the leaves of a tree, let water cool your hands and face. Turn within to that place of tranquillity. Leave your fears and worries there. Surrender them to the light inside you. Remember, you are never alone."

Wendy nods tearfully.

After a while I say softly, "I feel you have never lost sight of the guy who gave you the suitcase."

"No." She blows her nose. "I just forget to remember."

She sighs deeply and takes her drawing book out of her yellow bag.

"Mustn't forget to take that suitcase to my next appointment in the hospital."

"I suggest you leave it in the car," I reply, looking at the drawing she has put in front of me.

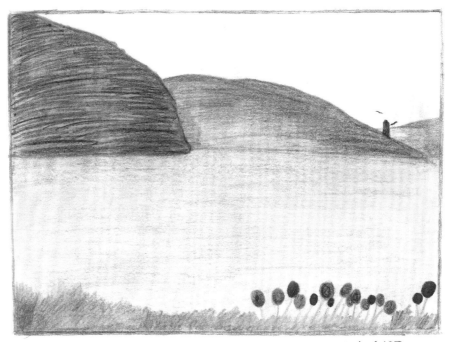

2 April '95

Her drawing: a dark lighthouse, purple and red flowers growing near the edge of the water.

"The light is out. That's how I sometimes feel. This bird has come back from the land to be with the other bird and they're together again."

"The sea looks very calm."

"Yes. Maybe I need to remember that God might be in every drop of water after all."

I count the flowers. There are sixteen flowers and seventeen stems. One flower has fallen off. I reflect on how all this is directly beneath the dark lighthouse.

About ten days later I receive a phone call from Wendy. She has left school and plans to study by correspondence again. "I had to try it. I know now that everything's changed forever. I want to be honest with myself and be who I really am. Time is precious. My body needs much more rest. And sunsets."

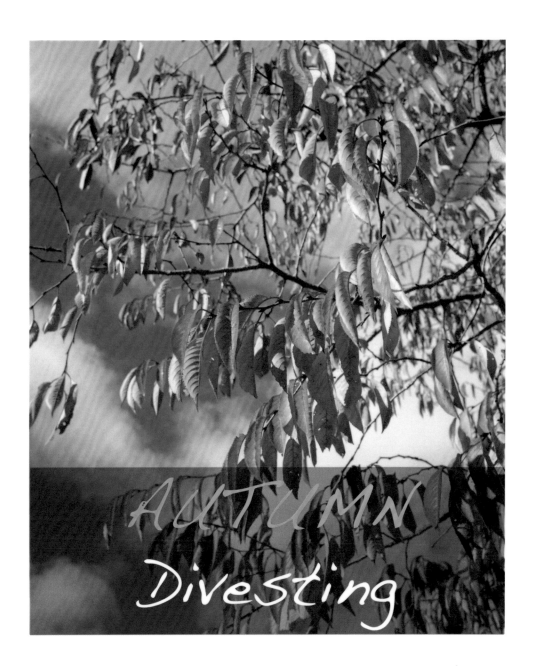

AUTUMN
Divesting

May 1995

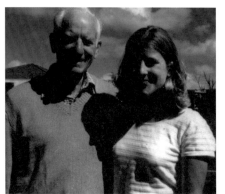

With her granddad Ted …

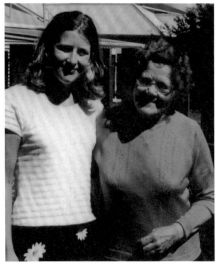

… and her nana Joan.

"THIS IS YOUR LUNCH TODAY." Wendy arrives carrying a precariously placed punnet of strawberries on top of her books and backpack. Her favourite purple boots complement a multi-coloured sweater and jeans. We chat about movies and our dogs and savour the strawberries.

"How are you?" I sort through the reports in Wendy's file.

"Not all that bad. Do you have the results of the x-ray? My cough's annoying."

"Yes, here it is. The lungs are clear, but there are enlarged lymph glands in the mediastinum, which is in your chest between your lungs." I demonstrate using my own body. "These glands can cause pressure and irritation, hence the cough."

"So I assume I just have to put up with it?"

"Well, we sometimes prescribe prednisone, but I'd rather start with some cough mixtures."

"Okay, hopefully it won't get worse."

I weigh her. "I see you've lost some weight."

"Wait till Lisa gets back and we start our chocolate binges again. Those kilos will come running back, maybe. My diet's too severe. And might I bring your attention to these scales? What are they, antiques? You sure they still function?"

"I won't hear a word against my 50-year-old scales," I laugh. "Is Lisa coming back earlier?"

"She's thinking about it. I told her about my glands and school and she heard me coughing and got upset. I said I was fine, but I'm not sure if she believed me."

"Are you fine?"

"Hmm. No, not always. I keep thinking about your suitcase story. And you'll be happy to know my suitcase is more open than closed at the moment. I feel much better after a good cry. I hope I'm not running out of tears."

"Hardly, I have been told the supply is infinite."

"What a relief."

"You're spending a lot of time by yourself. Do you see your grandparents?"

"I visit them often, especially now that Lisa's away and Mum and Dad are both working full-time. We drink tea and play games, and we walk to the lighthouse. I think they feel so helpless, not being able to make things 'better'. The other day Nana said: 'If only it was possible to swap places'."

"The perfect gift of life."

She opens her drawing book. "Here is number one."

"Ah, the first picture without a frame. Out in the open now."

"I hadn't even noticed that. Yes, I guess I am more open about my cancer and the way I choose to live my life."

There is a new sense of freedom in Wendy's drawing. At the same time she has drawn a large rock in the river, making travel treacherous; a barbed-wire fence with one of the poles fallen over; a flaxbush growing quite high and flowers in the middle. The river will flow downwards, ultimately merging with the ocean. Water merging into water again. I sense that in the picture, with the obstacle course of fence and flax, we're allowed to smell the flowers, but we have to be invited to share the song of her soul.

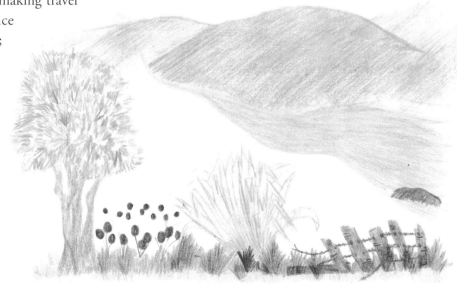

15 April '95

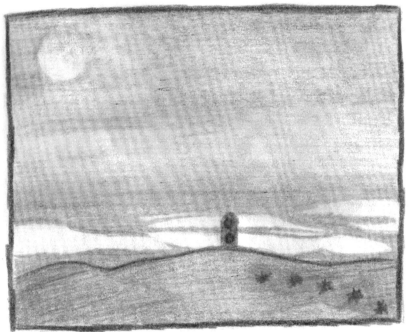

21 April
night-time

"I have another drawing, called 'night-time'."

I wonder, another lighthouse? A beacon? "Does it have a story?"

"Last time I went to the hospital they said it would be 'the end of the road' if I didn't accept treatment. It was awful. Later I walked along the beach. It was raining and there was a lot of wind. I watched the waves beating the sand and I suddenly felt so angry. I screamed a lot and I felt better afterwards. During the night I sat up and watched the clouds dancing in the light. The wind drove them along the sky while they swallowed up the moonlight.

And then a moment later the light was released again. I must have sat there for hours, I can't remember." She grins. "I must have danced as well. And then I drew this, early in the morning."

"Is it the end of the road?"

"No, it's not." She points at the little dots in the picture. "These five steps are my family and me. We form a path."

"Where are you in the drawing?"

She indicates the first dot. "That's me."

"So you're walking in front?"

"Yes."

Wendy is absorbed in her thoughts. "I am the closest to the light."

Her words seem to echo in my mind, slowly releasing a sense of infinity within. Finally Wendy turns another page.

"My last one."

I contemplate her drawing for a moment. "Tell me about the purple hills."

"For me the purple hills hold the nothingness, the silence."

She pauses and says softly, "They're still far away."

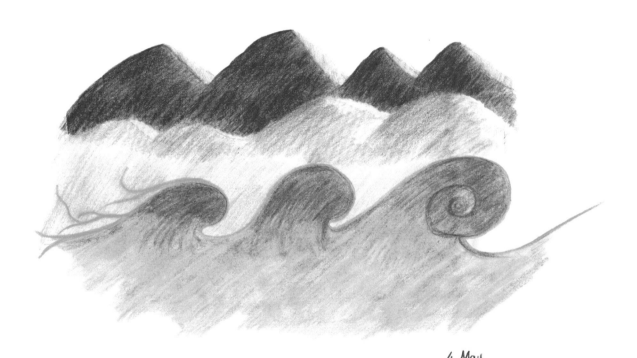

4 May

AFTER WENDY'S REGULAR VISIT to the Oncology Clinic I receive a letter:

24 July 1995

Dear Dr Rodenburg

I saw Wendy in clinic today with her father. I note that her weight has decreased by 10 kilos over the past seven months. She denies other symptoms of active Hodgkin's disease, but on examination there are palpable nodes in the right inguinal region and in the lower cervical regions, as previously noted.

I have again advised Wendy that in my opinion we should biopsy the inguinal node to confirm that it contains active Hodgkin's disease, and that in the very likely event of this being so, proceed to chemotherapy, initially with conventional three to four weekly cycles, but then high dose chemotherapy with peripheral stem cells. This would of course be a major undertaking, putting her life at risk and with no guarantee of success at the end, but in my opinion offers her the only prospect of long survival, perhaps equating to cure. For very understandable reasons Wendy has always been resistant to the idea of further treatment, and I would not seek to try and coerce her, but I have the feeling that time is beginning to run out, and if she loses much more weight she could get too sick for active treatment even to be an option. She has great confidence in you and finds it easy to talk to you, so I have suggested she do this quite soon.

[name]

Medical registrar, Oncology Unit
Wellington Hospital

Wendy walks into my room looking better then I expected.

"You got the letter?" she asks, as she throws her coat over the other chair.

"Yes, I just read it again."

"Well, I presume you want to 'discuss treatment options with me again'." She mimics the voice of one of her doctors.

"That's what's suggested by your specialist, so excellently voiced by you."

"The doctors are putting so much pressure on me. I hardly understand what they're talking about, but what I do know is that the treatment is quite dangerous. I could die during it, and nobody knows if it'll work or not."

"That's true. Anything can happen as a result of this treatment. It can affect other organs, infections can result, and the outcome's uncertain. It's the only treatment the medical profession can offer you at this moment, and I need to tell you there are some success stories as well."

"I know, and that's wonderful. But it's not the right treatment for me. I've thought about it again, but the answer is still no. Other people might have trust in the treatment, but I don't any more. I'm learning to trust my intuition, and my intuition tells me no."

"What about your parents, what do they think?"

"I know they're really worried. Dad's scared after talking to the doctors. He's reading a lot, trying to understand more about the treatment and procedure. Mum is very quiet, and Lisa has taken refuge in her diary. We had a family gathering the other night to talk about my cancer and what I want to do. They accept I need to make this decision by myself and they give me the freedom to do that."

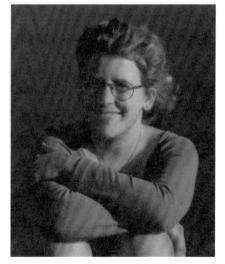

"Your family must be worried, scared and perhaps even angry. Do they share this with each other or do you talk about those feelings as a family?"

"Not really. I think all of us just try to get on with things and keep it normal, but of course it's bloody well not normal, is it? Not when you're 18 years old and the doctors tell you your time is running out. I wanted

> filled with anger and rage darkened
> clouds possess the sky threatening
> the land with an unruly downpour
> however
> the land feels no intimidation instead
> summons the rains with parched
> meadows and dehydrated riverbeds

to scream, 'How dare you say my time is running out?' I don't know whether I was more angry or scared."

I don't comment and she's meditative for a long moment.

"Oh, Rachel and Chris are getting married in October. It was brought forward because apparently I'm short on time. Everybody hopes I'll still be able to dance and get drunk."

We sit in the silence that follows humour when we're taken out of our comfort zone. I feel an unexpected and deep sadness.

"Do you feel that my time is running out?" She looks at me as if she knows the answer. "Do you think I should have the chemo?"

I deliberate. "I can't answer that. I can say as a doctor: you have a slight chance with chemo but the side effects can be horrendous. Is it worth taking the risk? I don't know."

She reaches for her coat and announces: "Well, I do know." There is utter conviction in her voice. "I have a lot more living to do."

Wendy leaves and I make a few notes. I gaze at the tree outside the surgery window. Bare branches reaching out towards the sun. A bird sings, resting, before taking flight again. I still feel sad.

It is good that next week I will spend two days with some colleagues who work in the same field. I need to talk about what's happening with Wendy and me.

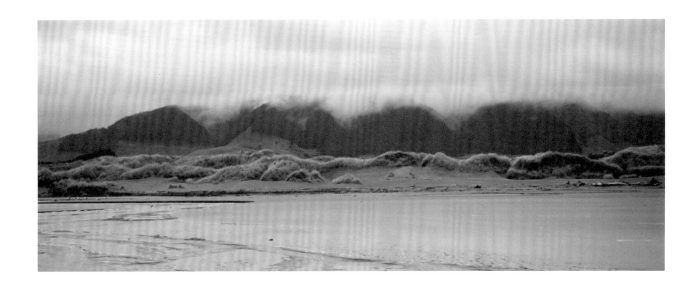

September 1995

WENDY STRIDES INTO MY ROOM with a bunch of daffodils and irises in her arms. She seems relaxed and tanned.

"These are for you. The frangipani didn't make it through the flight."

"They're gorgeous." I am truly delighted. "But what do you mean frangipani? And where did you get that tan?"

She is surprised. "I went to Fiji with Mum and Dad. I left a message with your nurse. Didn't you get it?"

"I got a message you were going away for a week to catch some sun. But she left Fiji out. I thought you were trying your luck in Golden Bay."

She flops into the green armchair. "It was nice to go away with Mum and Dad. We all slept a lot. I think we all really needed the break. I walked a lot along the beach, the colours of the sea are so exquisite. I got loads of sun because I only went inside to eat or sleep. Mind you, there were a few snacks at the pool side."

"You might be glad I've got such antique scales after all."

She burst out laughing. "We'll see. Truth comes in numbers, antique or not. Oh, I had a big surprise — Lisa arrived back from London and picked us up from the airport. It's so wonderful having my best friend in the same house again."

She digs into her bag. "I've got some drawings I did in Fiji, in between eating and sleeping."

Two palm trees, one short and sturdy, the other tall. "The short one is me."

"Not particularly a pushover, especially since the other tree seems to take the brunt of the wind."

13 August, Fiji

78

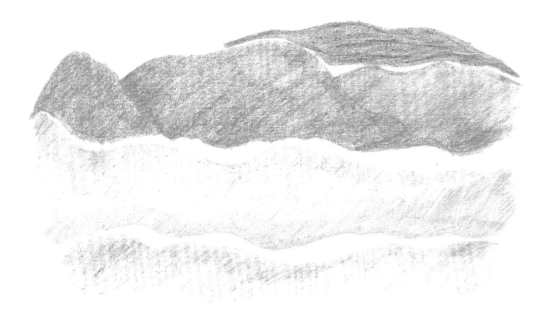

Wendy's face lights up, clearly pleased. "I have quite a few 'tall trees' in my life."

"And the purple hills?"

She smiles. "Yes. The purple hills and the sun going down behind them."

"When's your next hospital appointment?"

"Oh, it's coming up soon. I want to talk with you about that. I know they'll try to convince me to have more treatment, but I don't want it, no matter what happens."

"Wendy, you're aware that your cancer is active. Thanks to your lifestyle, diet, your creativity and the work you do with Raven, there's very slow progression, but there's progression nevertheless. At the moment you have chosen quality of life and refuse any invasive treatments. If this is your final choice, you need to discuss this with the doctors in the Oncology Clinic. Because you don't want any intervening therapy any more, they might very well refer you to the hospice for ongoing care. Do you know about the hospice, Wendy?"

"I've heard the name, but I don't know much about it. I thought it was a place where people go to die."

"People often have the wrong impression of a hospice. Most people think when their doctor refers them to a hospice, this is probably 'the beginning of the end'. But that's not true. It's a place with an emphasis on living rather than dying, and on health rather than disease. It's about living in the moment and at the same time accepting death as an inevitable outcome.

"The emphasis is on maximum and optimal symptom control. And hospice-trained doctors and staff are very skilled at achieving that. It often creates a quality of life which in itself often creates quantity — more time. It is treatment in a way, but the focus is not on a cure. And the patient is always part of the decision-making."

"What kind of decisions?"

"Well, for instance, decisions about medication, diet, and sometimes admission for rest, pain relief, or a break for the caregiver. The focus is on making you more comfortable, hopefully on all levels: the physical, mental, emotional and spiritual. People can enjoy life and find a purpose in their day-to-day living. There's a lot of emphasis on creativity and you can attend art classes there as well."

"Are the classes only for patients in the hospice?"

"No, it's primarily for outpatients, people who are under hospice care but are at home."

"That's what I want."

"You might need one of your 'talking circles' at home."

"Yeah, I need to think about how I'll tell them, they might have the same idea as I did about a hospice."

I weigh up my words. "I want to ask you a question. We are talking about *your* life, talking about *your* possible death. How do you feel?"

She looks out the window, deep in thought. "Right now I'm not sure how I feel. I'm not scared. I feel safe here with you. I know whatever I ask you, you'll always be honest with me. I never feel like a patient here."

I'm moved by her words.

"I feel I can be me here, just Wendy. I know I have cancer, I'm a woman with cancer, but I'm always Wendy here. You allow me to say how I really feel. I have to be careful, there's not many people I can really be myself with."

I agree. "Sometimes people don't know how to respond."

"That's right, and it makes me sad. I start doubting myself and I don't want to feel like that."

"Believe in yourself. Hold on to that love."

"I do, it's my lifeline. I won't allow cancer to grow into my heart."

A few days later I receive a copy of the referral letter to Mary Potter Hospice.

29 September 1995

Medical Director
Mary Potter Hospice
Newtown

I am writing to ask if you would accept the ongoing treatment and care of Miss Wendy Potter. Wendy was diagnosed in 1991 with lymphocyte predominant Hodgkin's disease.

Over the last three to four months Wendy has gradually become a little more unwell. Her current symptoms are lethargy, requiring extra sleeping time in the afternoon, most days. She has shortness of breath on moderate exertion, associated with a persistent but dry cough, she has a small appetite and does experience the occasional vomit after episodes of prolonged coughing. She is however feeling at peace within herself. She is living at home with her family, and her sister has returned to live with the family. They are able to get out and around most days, and Wendy still continues to work part-time at a voluntary job in the Correspondence School Library.

What has become clear however, over the last few months is that Wendy, despite extensive discussions is adamantly against any further aggressive chemotherapy. She has been talking these issues through with Dr Hetty Rodenburg as well as with her family. She recognises that she will undoubtedly become more frail and more unwell, and that she will die, although the timing of this we obviously cannot predict.

At Wendy's request we make this referral for her ongoing care. She is clearly going to need more medical support over the next months, and in view of the terminal nature of her illness she would like to become familiar with your services and surroundings as soon as possible.

[name]

Medical registrar, Oncology Unit
Wellington Hospital

November 1995

WENDY ARRIVES, WITHDRAWN AND SAD. "Was that Lisa with you in the waiting room? Do you want her to come in?"

"No, it's okay, she's off to see a friend. I didn't feel like driving today."

"What's happened?"

She shows me her drawing. "That's me."

The hills are dark and the water flows freely, not confined any more, almost cascading down. "So many tears."

"Yes, and they keep coming."

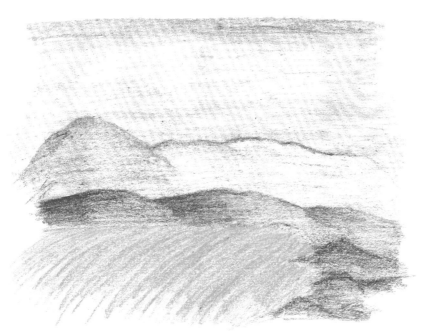

13 october

"Perhaps you're crying for all that you've never cried for before. The body never forgets."

She's crying now. "I don't have to know why I'm crying, do I?"

"No, my friend, tears have their own wisdom."

She is still teary. "Lots has happened. Rachel and Chris got married, earlier than planned because I was supposed to be half-dead." She laughs through her tears and

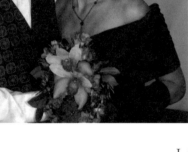

blows her nose. "Well, I'm not, and I had a good time. I ate plenty, drank a lot of wine and even managed to dance until late. Mind you, the next day I was a write-off, but it was worth it. Here's a photo of me and Reuben. Pretty good, eh?"

This is a testimony of life. Wendy's defiant smile, Reuben holding her close.

"You look lovely and certainly not half-dead. And …" I am rummaging through Wendy's file, "here is the letter from the hospice, Dr Rod MacLeod, with lots of positive comments about your health. And a three-month follow up. That's really good."

"Yeah, it's bizarre, the moment I'm referred to the hospice I'm feeling better."

"Well, it proves again, you are not a statistic."

For a while she doesn't speak. "Reuben and I have broken up."

I don't know what to say for a moment. "I'm really sorry to hear that. The photo tells a different story. You both seem so happy."

"We were. We are. It's not that we don't love each other. Reuben's finished Design School. He wants to go overseas, to the UK to work. I'll never be able to go with him. I have cancer and that's the truth and one day I will feel tired and shitty again and not want to go out. Even now I can't do it all the time. Reuben loves to go out and do things, late nights, long talks. He needs his freedom. I know very well that my chances of living a long life are very small. I'm coming to terms with that in my own way, very, very slowly. Reuben will probably disagree, but I think my illness and restrictions are sometimes quite hard for him."

"Did you make this decision?"

"We did talk about it together, but yes … I did. I've been thinking about it for a while."

"Reuben must be sad as well."

"Yep, we both are. But I know we'll always be friends. Ultimately I will need friends, not lovers."

After a while we turn to Wendy's drawings.

"That tree has a lot of blossoms."

"Yes, like my mother, she has so much to give, she's bending at the knees. Her whole life is around me and what I need."

I study the picture. The tree is laden with flowers and is bursting off the page.

"I wonder what's happening to the roots of these trees, I can't see them."

Wendy is deep in thought for a long time. "There's a lot to carry, I hope the roots are strong enough."

After she leaves, I write a few notes in her file:

> Wendy and her cancer central
> focus in this family.
> Relationship Janet-Cyril?
> How much energy is left for
> each other?

I reflect on the toll it takes on a family where a child has been diagnosed with cancer.

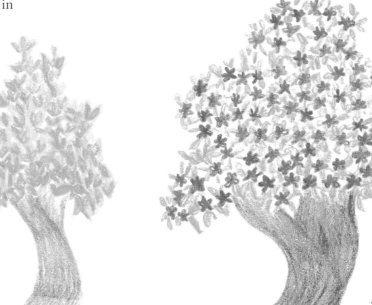

2 November

Studio 2005

I READ THROUGH SOME of my notes and journals and think about Wendy's next burst of energy at that time, her frequent outings, the little events she organised for the family, gaining some weight and living an almost 'normal' life. I remember talking about it with Janet at the time, explaining that it wasn't unusual.

Diseases like cancer hardly ever follow a straight line. There will always be fluctuations in the disease progression, with ups and downs on the physical as well as the emotional levels. It frequently plateaus, and for a while it might appear that the cancer has gone into remission.

Young cancer patients in particular adjust their activities to that level and can become quite active, enjoying life. Wendy was very aware of this stage of her cancer and used the extra energy to indulge in outings with friends and exploring Wellington's nightlife.

She wanted to come and see me very regularly from this point on.

January 1996

I CLOSE THE DOOR TO MY HOUSE and walk down the steps to the studio. It's a brilliant clear day. I see the sky reflected in the water of the birdbath.

The surrounding trees with their singing, winged inhabitants, the pansies and the white and pink roses all create a wonderful setting. Wendy prefers to meet here and I decided only to see her back in the surgery when she needs a physical examination or possible referral for tests.

"You look great, Wendy."

"Yep, I feel it. I'm less tired, my appetite's getting better, and even my cough's not so bad."

"What have you been up to?"

"The real question is, what has she not been up to?" Lisa, who is with her today, answers instead.

"I'm having a great time with Lisa. Still going out in the daytime, and some evenings as well."

Lisa cuts her off. "In the evening she prefers male company, although I'm still allowed to drive."

"Who's the favourite man at the moment?"

"I spend a lot of time with Richard. We've been friends for ages. He's fun and looks after me when I drink too much."

Lisa starts to laugh. "We'll call you some time when Wendy's on the dance floor. She's a sight to be seen and not always willing to come home either."

Wendy's not smiling any more.

"I know this won't last, but right now, I want to do something other than just 'being careful and working hard to stay healthy'. There are times I even forget I have cancer."

"How are things at home; how are your parents?"

Again, Lisa answers. "Mum and Dad were quite upset when the hospice was first mentioned. But I think they feel a little happier now, because as you know, Wendy started to feel better the moment she was referred to the hospice. I think all of us, Mum, Dad, Rachel to some extent, and me, we all live from day to day and try to keep a sense of normality. You really hold it all together, Wenz. If it weren't for your 'around the table' meetings, we might not talk at all."

Wendy opens her drawing book.

"You've drawn the sun so large here."

"Yes, this tree needs a lot of warmth and light. It has so much blossom."

I notice one branch of the tree is growing away from the main stem and some of its foliage is no longer visible; it has fallen off the page. The tree appears strong, but I wonder if the roots are deep enough to hold the tree up. I think back to the drawing she brought in last November of the two trees, neither of which had visible roots.

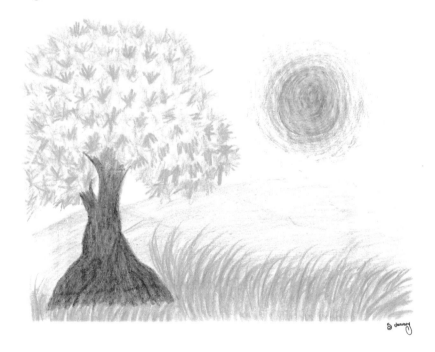

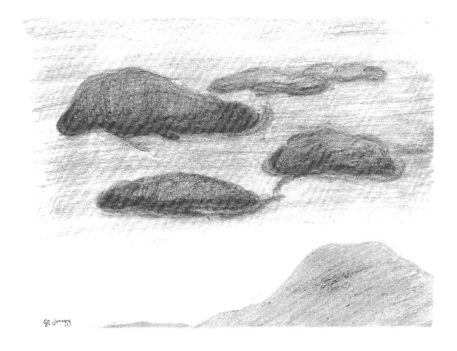

21 January

I study the setting sun in her second drawing, disappearing behind the green hills, not much land, a striking sky and four red clouds. For a moment my medical mind takes over and I wonder if the clouds have something to do with her developing cancer. Are they cancer cells, multiplying rapidly?

"Tell me about this drawing."

"This sun is slowly setting, slowly going down. But there's still lots of light. The sun throws its light out in the sky and covers and holds the clouds and paints them red."

Four members of her family, four clouds. Wendy's love for her family, strong enough to colour the clouds scarlet in a blue and orange sky. I happily shift from my logical, medical mind, wearing a white coat when registering cancer cells, to 'diagnosing' Wendy's four scarlet clouds.

February 1996

"THE OTHER NIGHT I had such a frightening dream. It reminded me of the hospital, the needles and treatments and not being in control. I couldn't get away."

"Tell me about it. I might be able to help."

"I hope so … I dreamt I was in a room in the hospital. There was a trolley, a bed. In the corner was a desk and on the desk was a file. I knew it was my file, my name was on it. It was about my life; it was about what's going to happen to me. On the other side of the room were instruments and things, drips, needles and there was a door. The door was closed. I was lying on the trolley and was so scared. I was scared that they might want to treat me again. And I didn't want it and I couldn't get out. When I woke up I was crying. I was so frightened. I can't stop thinking about it."

"Wendy, we can go through your dream together, would you like to do that? It's important you find 'the way out' and feel in charge again."

"Yes, I want to do that."

"We need to go on a journey. The journey starts in that same room, but before we go there we need to make sure that you feel safe. What do you need to feel safe? What do you need to take with you on the journey?"

Wendy is quiet for a while. "I take my crystal, the one I always hold in my hand when I meditate."

"Good, and perhaps you want to put a cloak around you as well. I want you to feel protected and safe."

There's no fear any more, only curiosity.

"Just sit comfortably and close your eyes. Now I want you to go back to that room. The room will be exactly how you saw it in your dream and you are lying on the trolley. I want you to come off the trolley. You're not tied down, and if you are, you can undo the straps. So step down and look around. In the corner is the desk with your file on it. Do you want to read that file, about your life, about your illness?"

"No, no, I don't want to know about that."

"Good. Can you see the door?"

"Yes."

"Is the door still closed?"

"Yes."

"Go to the door and open it … Have you opened it?"

"Yes."

"What do you see?"

"It's dark ahead of me, it's like a corridor, a tunnel. I don't know."

"Before you can go through a doorway you need to talk to the spirit of the door and ask for permission to pass. Ask if it has a message for you. Ask what you need to learn before you're allowed to go through the door, into the corridor."

Wendy is silent for a while before she answers.

"The spirit of the door tells me that doors are about freedom, that I'm not a prisoner, that the door is open. It's only my fear that creates a prison and keeps me hostage."

"Thank the spirit of the door and then walk on. Remember you're not alone, and the crystal will protect you. Just walk on and tell me what you see."

"It's becoming lighter. There's another door, no, it's like a gateway or a portal."

"Go through that portal, find what you need to learn and what the spirit of the portal can teach you."

"It's a gentle spirit, it's so kind to me. It tells me about courage, and about the gateways that lead us into other worlds."

"Again, thank the spirit and continue."

Wendy walks on. It's become her journey now. There are doors to be opened, there's light, there's darkness, she's turning corners, sometimes to the left, sometimes to the right. There are more gateways. She greets them, connecting easily. She asks for permission to move through. She becomes more and more relaxed. I watch her as I guide her on this path. She seems more peaceful, her breathing easy and slow.

The messages to Wendy are about letting go of fear. Fear is a state of mind that limits our ability to be free. There are messages about believing in love and in understanding that love is the essence of our being.

Her face changes until it literally radiates. "I'm standing in front of a garden, I've never, ever seen anything like this. Oh, this is so beautiful."

It's as if she's left my room. I see a body sitting in a chair, a very relaxed body, but the owner has really gone on a journey. Time stands still, there is only the experience of being here in this moment, in the now. All there ever is, there ever was, there ever will be. I still remember the feeling of peace, of infinite compassion, slowly enveloping me as I watch her.

After some time, almost thirty minutes, the doctor/counsellor in me returns and I start to consider several options for contacting Wendy in her undoubtedly celestial garden, and guiding her back to my cosy, but earthly room. The moment this thought enters my mind, Wendy starts to cough. It's one of those coughs which can last for up to a minute, and it causes Wendy to return with a jolt, an unexpected yet still delicate crash-landing back in her chair.

For quite a while she doesn't speak. Her face still radiates, something has changed. "I don't know how to describe what I've just seen, what I've just experienced, but I'll show you my drawing. I did this two days before my dream."

There is a garden full of flowers and colourful butterfly-like creatures.

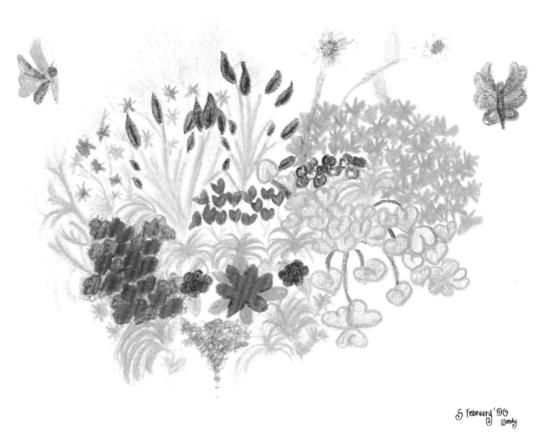

5 February '96
Wendy

"This is the garden where I've just been. I met them all."

"Who did you meet?"

"The little creatures, the ones who come to me in my dreams or when I meditate or when I'm scared. Here they are. There were butterflies and a dolphin and there was somebody else. A child. I met this child and I know who she is. She is me. I've given her a name — Starchild."

I've never seen Wendy so excited. Her face is soft, there is a golden glow like a beautiful full moon on a bright summer night.

After Wendy has left, I stay in the deep silence she has left behind.

I see Wendy later in the month and it's obvious her garden journey has been the beginning of another transformation.

"I've been back to my garden quite a few times, and I've had glimpses and experiences of other dimensions. It's hard to describe, but I feel so good, so safe and cared for. I know now I'm never alone."

"How do you get there?"

"Raven helped me to visualise the garden and the creatures and then I just 'go'. It's really easy, and it feels so normal to be there."

within the tenderness of peace
i close my eyes
and search for the garden in which
my starchild lies
i see her sleeping and who wakes
from her dreamland
with lovingness i hold her close in
the palm of my hand

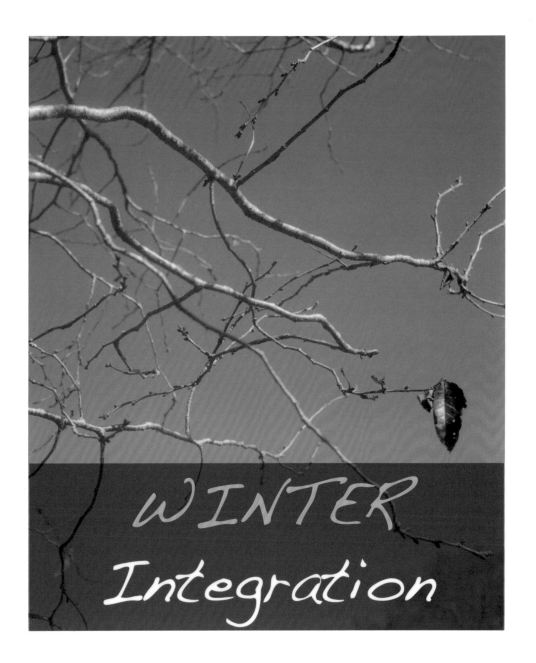

WINTER
Integration

March 1996

WENDY'S SHORT BURST OF ENERGY over the summer months is waning and she is forced to rest more and restrict her fun activities. Her recent experience during the dream session and her nana's death — she passed away a few weeks ago after a short illness — compel Wendy to spend a lot of time by herself.

"I'm often wondering, is there a purpose being here? What could be the purpose of my life?"

"Do you have any ideas?"

"My sense is it has something to do with feeling peaceful and content with life. Like Nana, always so kind and grateful for everything, generous and full of hope. She couldn't make my cancer better, but she sure knew how to make me feel better."

Wendy tells me how she feels Nana's presence sometimes. "I believe her spirit will continue Hetty. Her spirit cannot die."

Listening to Wendy I'm conscious of her growing awareness that life has no end, that death is a transition, a doorway through which we move into different realms of consciousness. She verifies this: "Death does not exist. I believe that my body will fall away and that my spirit, my essence will continue. I don't know where and how. But I know that my spirit is immortal."

"When you visit your garden, is the child you called your Starchild there?"

"Oh, yes, Starchild is always there, she makes me happy."

"Who is she?"

"It's not so easy to find the words for her. She's me, she's a part of me. She's free and is outside me and inside me. She is my constant companion."

"Do you feel now that she has always been a part of you?"

"Yes, she has always been with me, but now I've experienced her. Now I know she's always been a part of me."

She opens her book.

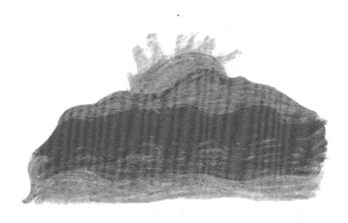

15 March

"That was a great day. I thought a lot about your bus story and all the different Wendys who are sitting in my bus. I like talking to them. I believe they give me inspiration and insights. I call them my stars."

"And what do the stars think about this?" I point at her drawing.

"It's the sun rising behind the purple hills. I feel the purple hills are what death is all about." She counts the rays. "Seven."

I'm mesmerised by her drawing. But what does it remind me of? I remember a diary in which I used to copy excerpts from texts from ancient India. "I have something I want you to read."

I go to my study and pull out some of my old diaries and within minutes I've found what I want. I give her the book, page open.

"This is what your drawing reminds me of."

> Even as darkness is dispelled by the rising sun, the world illusion is dispelled when the sun of infinite consciousness arises in the heart. He who knows that which alone is worth knowing, transcends all coming and going, birth and death.

Wendy reads it a few times to herself. When she looks up she has tears in her eyes and says softly: "I don't understand it all but I feel like I'm being held in a bubble of joy."

"Perhaps this is not about understanding, perhaps this is about the experience of joy."

When Wendy leaves, she assures me she is fine. "I'll go and sit on the beach for a while before driving back to Wellington. Might have a little chat with Nana. She knew about joy."

I write some notes, remembering her words about death. I can still see her drawing in front of my eyes.

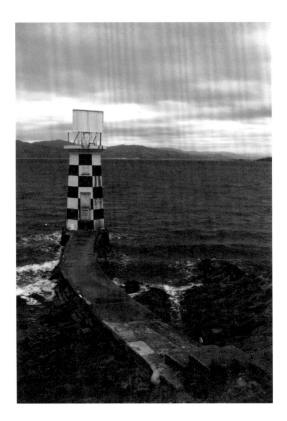

Wendy's favourite lighthouse,
Point Halswell, Wellington Harbour.

April 1996

"BEEN TO THE HOSPICE, they've put me on some prednisone. Have to go back in three weeks."

"Good."

Wendy puts her cup of lemon zinger tea down. "I'm thinking a lot about death. About my own death. Death, or perhaps it is called dying, feels such a slow process. I die a little every day. And I never know what bit will be taken away. It feels like a sculptor chipping away at me, bits falling on the ground, like little pieces falling away out of my life."

"What are some of those pieces, those small deaths?"

"Things I can't do because of my tired body. My sadness that I will have to say goodbye to all and everything." After a pause, "My future seems to be only in the now."

"Perhaps the now is really all we have."

"Sometimes I feel I have no control at all."

"You will have control and you will always have choices. You can decide how to be and how to perceive the world. Nobody can take that away from you. Only you will make the decision how to respond to your illness; only you can choose how to be on the path ahead of you. Do you allow yourself to be filled with fear, or do you trust you'll never be alone? Will you be anxious or will you have faith in the power of this universe to heal the hearts of your family?"

"You're right. I will always have choices, won't I?"

"Yes, you will. Think of the bird in your drawing, flying to the lighthouse. Become that bird and fly to the lighthouse where the waves are crashing against the walls, but inside it's safe and warm, like coming home again."

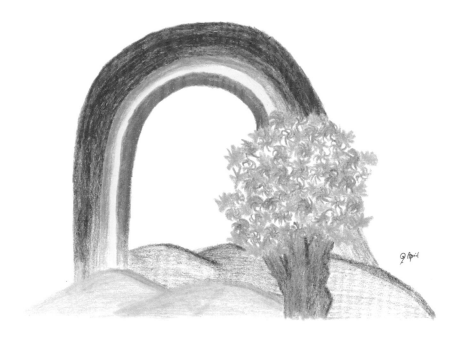

Wendy has drawn green and purple hills. A beautiful rainbow creates a doorway to another world. There's a flowering tree and the bottom part and roots are not visible. I notice four branches. On the right side a branch has been cut off.

"Lots of flowers on that tree."

"Yes, autumn hasn't arrived yet."

She turns the page, to another drawing.

"This was in my dream and I couldn't wait to start drawing it when I got up: a star within a star."

"There's your seven again. The number of perfection and completion."

"Good, perhaps it holds my destiny," she laughs, "matches my 7-7-77 birthday."

I'm drawn to the white five-pointed star in the centre and wonder when it will be ready to expand and fill the space with its light.

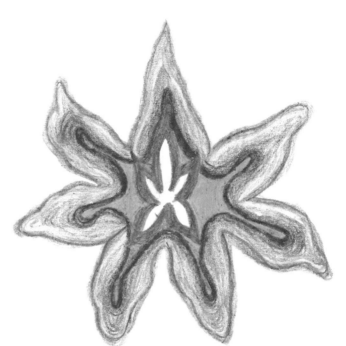

15 April

i close my eyes
from now and then
and become a shining star
or sit within my pearly cloud
up in the sky so far
or else i stay and simply sit
with my company
i sit and be all that i am
happily being one

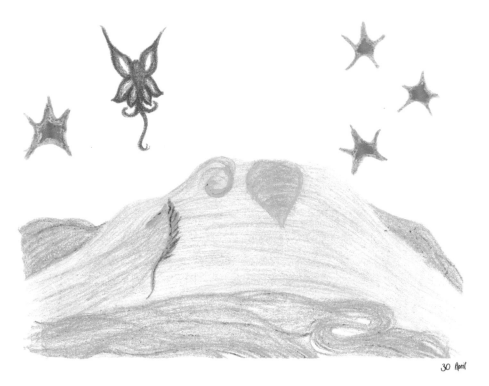

30 April

May 1996

"I'M STILL SHORT OF BREATH, especially at night and when I walk uphill."

"Are you taking the Dexamethasone prescribed by the hospice?"

"Yes, I think I'm not as bad as when I saw the doctor, but I get frightened sometimes. It's like there's water in my lungs instead of air. Do you think that's how I will die? Drowning in that water, not able to breathe?"

She is so vulnerable and I wish I could tell her not to worry, that all will be fine. But I can't. "I don't know how you will die. I do know that we will always be there for you, to help you and do whatever we can."

"A few nights ago I couldn't sleep and did some drawings." She reaches into her bag, opens her drawing book and places it on the desk.

Is it an island? Some vegetation? A starry night?

I turn the drawing ninety degrees. I can see a face now, just above the water.

"Tell me about this beautiful creature in the sky surrounded by the four stars."

"That's me, and that's me as well," pointing at the face in the water. "That's how the world sees me and knows me, as Wendy, but that's only a small piece of who I am. Most of who I am is submerged." She points at the little creature. "That's where I am, looking at myself. The stars are my family, my father is next to me and on the other side are Mum and Rachel and Lisa."

I study the drawing again and realise her face is entirely above the water, her mouth and nose free to breathe.

"It might sometimes feel as if there is water right inside your lungs, but you will never drown in it, you will always be able to breathe, like the Wendy in the picture."

She gives me a cheeky grin. "Should have known that — after all, I did the drawing."

She looks at her hands and plays with her bracelet. "I dream often of Nana, and I know she keeps an eye on me. I miss her a lot but I'm not sad about her any more."

"What are you sad about?"

"Giving up my dreams. Like travelling overseas with friends and falling madly in love. I had dreams of studying, perhaps being a writer, I don't know. Perhaps having children. I have to let my dreams go, one by one."

I'm moved by her courage and determination as she slowly unties the knots, letting her dreams float away into infinity.

"You do have to let go, and I know it's hard and it hurts a lot." Wendy blows her nose. "For the journey you're embarking on you have to travel light."

"Travel light?"

It starts to rain and I get up to close the window. "Yes. You are deciding what to take with you on this journey: what to pack in your suitcase and what to leave behind. On this trip you don't want to take too much luggage, particularly nothing you don't want or need any more. So it's really about how to 'travel light'. Not such an easy task. You can't take the precious treasures of the past and the hopes and visions of a future. You have to leave them behind. In a way, travelling light means that you have no luggage at all."

Wendy leans back on the couch. "Empty-handed, you mean. Well, getting through customs won't be a problem." We both laugh.

"We all have many stories, some complete, some unfinished, and some we wish we could rewrite and give a happier ending."

"I have a few unfinished stories in my bag. I'm not sure about the happy endings."

"And that's all part of it. Some stories never end, and others go out of print. One day you'll leave behind your legacy of love and of sadness, like the two sides of a coin. You need to keep some space in your travel bag, because you will carry that love and sadness as well. You have enough time to rearrange, to pack and unpack. I know you will ultimately travel very light."

I walk Wendy to her car, and just before she leaves she says: "I often think of your stories, like God and the little personal suitcase he gives us and how to use it and keep it very tidy. Today sounds a lot easier."

She sees my inquisitive look and adds:

"Well, if I want to, I can just throw the whole lot out."

I'm still laughing when I wave goodbye.

June 1996

JANET AND WENDY have just returned from a short holiday in Sydney. The first thing I notice is Wendy's blazing red hair.

"I dyed it again yesterday. It's my favourite colour."

"And certainly a statement not to be missed."

She has a twinkle in her eye when she asks, "Really? What kind of a statement?"

"Well, let me see, isn't it Raven who calls you 'She who must be obeyed?' I think that just about sums it up."

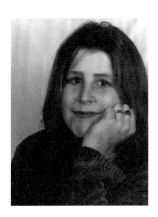

Wendy laughs. "I love my time with her. We're busy 'travelling' and discovering the universe."

"I'm sure the universe is discovering you as well. How was Sydney?"

"Great. We did the shops and arcades and saw *Phantom of the Opera*. Went on a harbour cruise and ate heaps."

"Any time to sleep?"

"Oh yes, our days were planned around my compulsory rests. The nights weren't particularly restful, because Mum snored and I coughed. We'd pushed the beds together in our room so we could sleep next to each other. Oh — I've got to tell you about the white fluffy towels in the hotel. I'm afraid they might never be the same again. You see, I'd dyed my hair just before we left and unfortunately put a little too much dye in, so every morning after my shower, the bathroom was like the Red Sea!"

"I don't think they'll want you back in a hurry."

"I don't think so." In an instant she becomes quite serious. "In fact, I doubt I'll be able to go anywhere any more."

She passes me her diary, the page open on 7 June. "I wrote this the other day. It's easier if you read it, you'll understand. I need to talk with my family because they need to know how I feel."

"Thank you."

Her handwriting is precise and small. Some daisies underneath?

"I hope they will understand how I feel. Sometimes it's difficult to find the right words."

"Stay with it. Those words and insights will come to the surface, like little bubbles full of wisdom rising from a dark ocean floor."

She reaches for her bag and takes out her purple drawing book.

"I did this the other night when I couldn't sleep."

Her drawing has soft colours and is centred in the middle of the page. An unfolding flower? Slowly revealing what's been hidden?

"Tell me about this blue-purple dot in the centre."

"I think that's where I go in my dreams, I feel safe there. After I finished the drawing I slept like a log. Lisa woke me up in the morning with a cup of tea. I think the tea was just an excuse, she was getting worried about my long sleep."

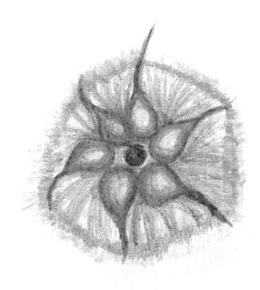

8 June

7 June

I feel like I really need to write down some of my thoughts before I can share them with my family.
I know from inside of me there is a lot of change. Many changes; some are what I think are truly beautiful because I see myself in places of comfort and love and others I sometimes feel are of loss. With these i do feel sad because it is part of me that is leaving. Then I think of the other pieces of me which will never fade or leave anyone. To me, every day is truly as it dawns and that is what I live it too. I have something around me all the time that helps me to be okay, my family. I want them to understand as best they can how I'm feeling. I want to be with them. I never want them to think I am giving up because I will never ever give up on living. I don't want to escape my life. I have so many treasures of love from each of them
The cancer I know, will never go away and I ask for help to be comfortable and supported.
I love you all so very much
now and always

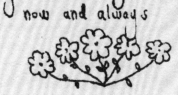

Later in the month I receive a letter from the hospice. Wendy did find the right words.

13 June 1996

Just a note to let you know that I met with the Potter Family (Wendy/ her parents, sisters and brother-in-law) on Tuesday 11 June 1996 and I was really privileged to be part of what was a remarkable family discussion.

Wendy talked about her feelings of huge sadness that had developed since she came back from Australia and the impression that she has that things are deteriorating for her. She wanted her family to know that she wasn't 'giving up' and this provided a wonderful opportunity for some very open discussion.

I talked about the availability of the Family Support Team to any or all of the family. I am sure that they may take this up at some point but at the moment they seem to be coping remarkably well with what is clearly a very sad situation.

The arrangement is now as before that Wendy will continue to see you, but I would obviously be happy to be involved at any time in the future.

With best wishes

Yours sincerely

Dr Rod MacLeod
Medical director

July 1996

GREY SKIES FULL OF RAIN and low-hanging mist hold the hills in a gentle embrace. Wendy walks through the garden towards the studio, her brightly coloured clothes a sharp contrast to the day's grey mantle — and my own black trousers and jersey.

She seems relaxed and doesn't seem to be coughing as much.

"Those cortisone tablets really helped. I sleep much better, my cough is less and I'm not so tired any more, finally. Life is really not too bad. There's always something to laugh about, especially with Lisa. I'm even baking my favourite muffins again. Sometimes I go to the park and sit on the bench there. I listen to the birds singing in the trees and watch the leaves changing colours."

"How are your mum and dad, and Lisa and Rachel? I know it must be so hard for them."

"Everyone's trying to be brave and they're not talking about it, but of course that's all that is on their minds. I know how sad they are, I can tell by Mum's face when she's been crying. I don't see Rachel that often. She is busy with her work and she has Chris. Lisa and I talk, like we've always done. She writes a lot in her journal, that really helps her. Yesterday she told me that it feels like the start of a waiting game."

"Does it feel like a waiting game for you?"

"No, not really. It's different for me, I'm not waiting. I'm much more trying to be present every moment."

"And your dad? How's he?"

"I think Dad's angry with the whole world. He must feel so desperate at times and of course angry. Angry with the world, the doctors and perhaps with himself for not being able to 'fix' his daughter."

"And the awful truth is he cannot fix you."

"I think I'm the son he never had. We've had such special times together, like our four-wheel driving, and the time we went to the Hippocrates clinic."

"Does he talk to his friends?"

"Yes, he has a few good mates, I think."

"And how's your mum?"

"She's trying hard to make it easier for me, but I know she often cries. Mum and I often talk, we've always been close. When I was little and sick, she'd often read me stories and stroke my back. She must've spent many sleepless nights with me."

"And what about you? How is Wendy?"

"Sad. Sometimes it almost overwhelms me, it hurts so much. I try to stay with it, really feel it, until that pain moves away. I don't feel angry or scared, not at the moment anyway."

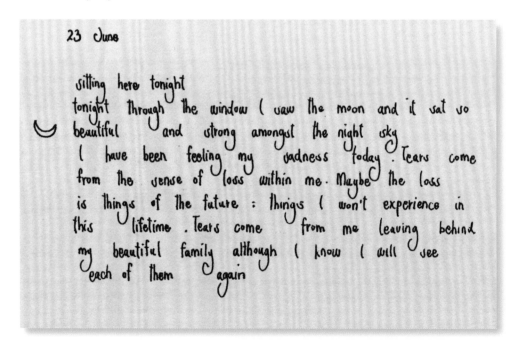

23 June

sitting here tonight
tonight through the window I saw the moon and it sat so beautiful and strong amongst the night sky
I have been feeling my sadness today. Tears come from the sense of loss within me. Maybe the loss is things of the future : things I won't experience in this lifetime. Tears come from me leaving behind my beautiful family although I know I will see each of them again

"I'm worried about my family. As you said, I'm the key player and everything does seem to revolve around me. I talk with each of them by themselves, but I don't think they talk to each other. I feel there's no willingness to share. I know that Mum and Dad aren't very close any more and perhaps my illness has something to do with it, but for quite a long time they've been drifting apart. Since my diagnosis it seems that it's me that holds them together. Everyone tries to stay normal for me."

"Does that upset you?"

She nods sadly.

"They must feel so lonely sometimes."

"When I'm not around any more …"

"What will happen then?"

"Everything might fall apart, I guess. It's strange because there is so much love, especially for me, and you'd think that if you're capable of feeling love, expressing love, that couldn't happen."

"I think relationships are hard work. We need to be able to communicate, to connect with each other. To feel safe to express whatever we feel and trust that the other will listen and not walk away or become defensive. And, as you said, have the willingness to share and be vulnerable. Love is a multicoloured coat and you have to wear it, you can't hang it in the cupboard. And that means it sometimes needs to get dirty."

"I like that! I must remember it."

She takes her coat off the chair. "I'll help them to prepare for what's ahead."

"You will be able to help them, but you can't take away their pain and sadness. You can't mend a broken heart, Wendy."

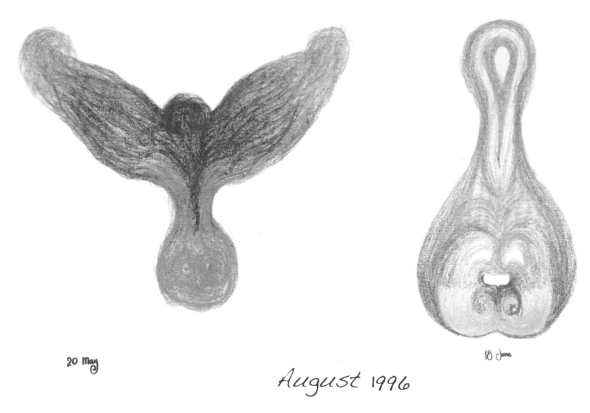

20 May

18 June

August 1996

WENDY SHOWS ME her last five drawings, all done between 20 May and 15 July.

Her pictures are intricate expressions of the many transformations taking place deep inside her. I am witness to the language of her soul.

"Is there a story?"

"It feels like I'm on a journey, going deep into the forest. There are clearings where the light streams in, and I can see blue sky among the treetops. I feel such calm and peace, no thinking, no questions, I'm just happy to be there. The pictures are 'the light breaking through'."

"That's a beautiful portrayal. Are you able to stay in that forest?"

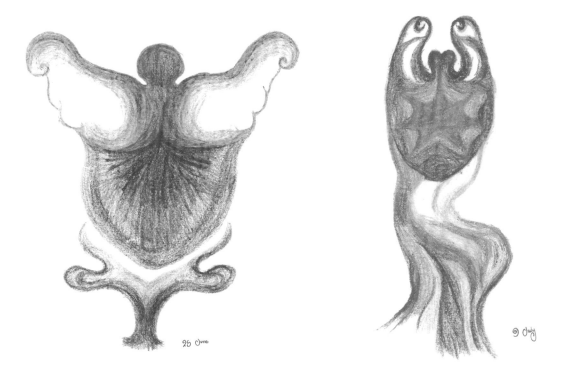

"No, I can't, but I'm learning to find the way back. Sometimes my mind wants to understand and becomes the guide in that landscape, and that's when I get lost."

For a moment I study Wendy's pictures with medical eyes. They remind me of photographs and drawings in my anatomy books of the reproductive system. Of the ovaries, the uterus, the umbilical cord. I've always imagined and experienced the concept of dying, of death, as a birthing process where ultimately the soul is released to continue its journey into consciousness.

"There's my star again." Wendy points at her fourth picture, on 9 July. A seven-pointed star confined within a purple enclosure.

"Yes, it's still inside."

"When I die my star will be free again."

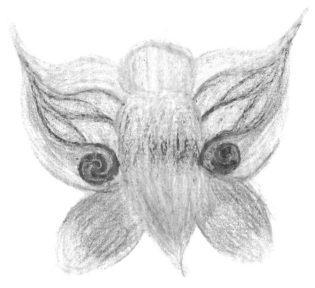

15 July

"What does freedom mean to you?"

"It's my ultimate destination. That's where 'home' is."

I feel I'm in the presence of a wise old soul who has taken temporary refuge in a young female body. "Tell me about this one," I finally say, pointing to the last one, drawn on 15 July, of a little yellow-winged creature.

"Oh, that was a really good morning, the sun was shining and I felt sort of playful and free."

"Free again."

I turn again to her drawing dated 9 July. It just might represent the earthly coloured umbilical cord still connected to and holding the body of the seven-pointed star — the soul. That connection looks strong to me and I wonder if Wendy's still got quite some time ahead of her.

One week later Wendy makes a quick visit to the surgery. "Guess what? Me and Lisa and Rachel are going to Rarotonga for a week! We're leaving in three days. I need a prescription for a Ventolin inhaler."

I notice her breathing is a little wheezy and I examine her. "Not too bad. Use your inhaler three to four times daily, then you won't have any problems flying. Are you looking forward to having time with your sisters?"

"I really hope by having this time together, sharing lots of things and having fun, it'll create a closeness between Rachel and me."

I write out the prescription as Wendy talks about her sisters.

"I was ten or eleven when I appointed myself as Lisa's shadow. Can't remember if it was mutually agreed, but Lisa dragged me along with great tolerance. We have similar personalities, we often think alike."

"And Rachel?"

"I love Rachel and we do get on, especially now, but we're not that close. I

Lisa and Wendy.

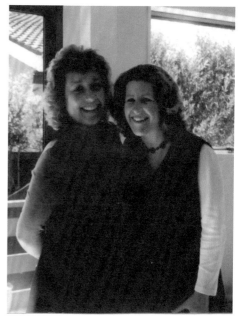

never really missed that because I had Lisa, and besides Rachel's seven years older and had her own friends. We had a lot of little fights and arguments, I remember, and poor Lisa was in the middle. Rachel must've felt left out sometimes, not only because of Lisa but because I was always sick with asthma and eczema, and being the youngest I got a lot of attention. I still do of course."

"When one child gets ill in a family, the attention goes off the other siblings. It's never a judgment on parents or caregivers, there's simply not enough energy left to nurture the whole family."

"Yes, and Rachel left home to live with Chris not long after I was diagnosed."

I hand her the prescription. "Let's hope you'll have a great time together among the sun, sand and coconuts."

Early September 1996

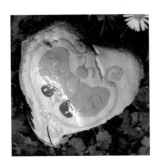

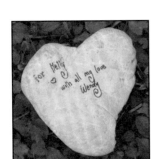

WENDY IS BEAMING when she walks into the studio and gives me a smooth grey stone with a butterfly painted on it.

"I know your passion for butterflies, and this will always remind you of me."

The stone is in the shape of a heart. "It's beautiful," I say, touched by her gift. "A new heart for the doctor."

"I found it in the forest and knew it was for you."

I read the words on the back, 'For Hetty, with all my love, Wendy'.

I give her a hug. "Thank you. This will be my special stone. How was Rarotonga?"

"We had a really good time and it was lovely, but I'd hoped for long talks and more closeness with Rachel. It didn't happen and I'm a little sad about that."

"Yes, you had great expectations. It's important to remember that your illness creates different realities for each member of your family."

"What do you mean?"

"Well, there's your reality, and nobody will really know, or feel what it's like for you to live with cancer. Nor will anybody really know what it's like for your mum and dad to have a daughter with cancer. And the same applies for Lisa and Rachel. Have you heard the saying, 'You don't know how somebody feels until you walk in their moccasins?' I think it's very true. Rachel's always had a different relationship with you, from the one you've had with Lisa, not that close, not that involved, not the same trust and bond. But she loves you, it's just expressed in different ways, on different levels and with different intensity."

"Yes, I do know she loves me. I guess I just need to respect that it's different."

"A relationship doesn't suddenly change when someone gets ill."

"I know, I can only change myself."

There are three more drawings.

An angel reaches out to a star. Is it an embrace of soul and spirit? I notice that the star is still encased. Not free yet.

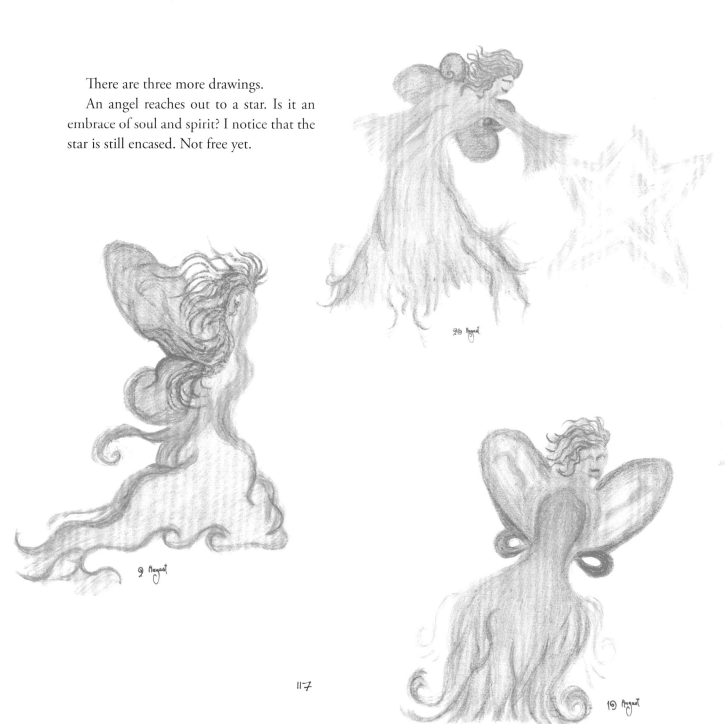

20 August

here i am ..

sitting in my bedroom while outside the sun sets into the
    nighttime and the winds blow
all day i have been feeling separate from everything and
anyone and very very tired
i have had the sensation of being very small , all i
want to do is be a little bundle
i feel very a lone and i'm hurting inside , myself
keeps on visiting the land of tears and i
have to go there and be within the earth and
trees and flowers so that my own garden can grow
i ask for harmony after my tears but somewhere
with them , when they surface , there is already
comfort
i know im okay and always will be
i know of beautiful love that surrounds me
i know my lovelight glows and is free
today my heart was aching which happens sometimes
but now i feel more quiet inside , more settled
        love you

She picks up her diary. "I wrote this on the same day as my third drawing, on the 26th of August."

"Is the land of tears a sad place to visit?"

"No, the sun shines there as well. I can get upset and feel very much alone, and yet at the same time I have this awareness that whatever is happening now, and whatever will happen in the future, I'll be okay. Do you understand what I mean?"

"Yes, I think so …"

Wendy interrupts. "You might even have another metaphor for me."

I pull a face. "I might just have one, an aeroplane this time."

"I need an aeroplane for all the suitcases I have been given for my journey."

We laugh.

"You see, Wendy," I point at her angel picture, "to fly and be free, wings are essential. It's like your bird and the angels. Or an aeroplane. Imagine you're in the pilot's seat. You have access to the instruments, you're in control. That's the place where you want to be. Where you need to be."

We talk about the wings of opposites. How there's the wing of birth and the wing of death, of laughter and of tears, of joy and despair, of love and fear, night and day, health and disease, spring and autumn.

I explain how these wings can also have different names like the 'known one' and the 'unknown one'. How we identify with the known one, we even give it a name, like Wendy. That wing encompasses our humanness, our efforts, our choices, our determination to reach our goals. The achievements and disappointments, the losses and gains, the mountains and valleys of life. The wing of doing, the wing of effort.

I describe the other wing, the unknown one; for most of us, a mystery. How it holds the answers to questions like: *Who am I? What is my purpose in this life? Is there life after death? Is there a God, a creator? Who created this universe?* A wing of divine wisdom and infinite loving. The wing of being, the wing of grace.

"To fly this plane isn't always easy. It's a delicate balance between trust and effort. Often we invest our power, our expectations of life, our faith and trust only in the wing of our human resources. And gradually we lose sight of grace. We don't even notice that we are really going out of balance. And for a while it seems to work and we fill our suitcases and carry them on board. In our need for security, we attach ourselves to material wealth and create a belief system around it. Finally we invest in refusing to see death as an inevitable part of life, and procrastinate perpetually, instead of investing any time in exploring the other wing of our plane. But then a crisis enters our life."

"Like cancer."

"Yes, like cancer and other life-threatening situations. Death, severe loss, human conflict or natural disasters. It's as if the wind beneath our wings has been taken away and we're afraid of crashing. Our beliefs and illusions of constancy and immortality are challenged, and we feel lost and scared. We wonder what to believe in, what to do, how to be, who to trust and what to put our faith in. The gods we worshipped and believed in, the gods of knowledge, wealth and technology, don't seem to have the answers any more."

"Yes, that's how I felt, their answers were no longer the right ones for me."

"Often life-threatening illnesses like cancer force us to explore the unknown. We need humility and sincerity in our plea for help. We need courage to look at our overfilled suitcases … we might even entertain a willingness to travel lighter."

I can see it's familiar territory I'm describing. "When you're in that pilot seat you will experience both wings as one. Then you can feel sad or scared, and at the same time trust in a power beyond our understanding." I lean back in my chair. "Well, this was rather a long flight."

"But it's given me the view I needed." She gets her long black coat from the chair and puts it on.

"That's a warm and cosy coat."

She grins. "This is no weather to travel light, Hetty."

Late September 1996

A KALEIDOSCOPE OF COLOURS greets me: red hair, blue dungarees, yellow top and big purple lace-up boots that walk Wendy effortlessly into my studio.

I give her a hug. "You look stunning, as usual. All the colours of the rainbow."

"Thanks. I feel pretty good. Hence my early rising, and *voilà!*" She opens her bag and puts freshly baked muffins on the table.

Enjoying her peppermint tea, Wendy casually mentions, "I'm preparing my funeral service, the cremation, the places I want my ashes to go to."

This matter-of-fact statement takes me completely by surprise. "I see," is all I manage to reply. No exception to Wendy's determination to make her own decisions, I think. There's no mistaking this is still her life.

She notices my surprise. "It's really important for me to make decisions about what'll happen with my body. It's part of my preparation for death."

"You're right. Do you feel scared, organising all this?"

"I have moments when I'm very scared of what's ahead, of what's going to happen to my body. I'm scared of dying, I suppose. But I'm not scared of death. I don't know in what form or state, but I know I'll continue. When my body dies I'll be free."

"It might still take a while."

"Yes, I know. But I feel it will be around Christmas."

Once again I stare at her in astonishment. It's quite rare that patients tell me their expected departure date, and certainly not in such a calm and matter-of-fact way!

"Christmas? Well, let's see. Death has its own time, not a minute too early and not a minute too late. You might think you're in charge of that time, but are you?"

Wendy listens politely, but I have a strong feeling she's not very open to amendments to her itinerary. We talk a bit about her medications. I ask again how her family's coping. She reiterates that they talk individually, but still not much as a family.

"I guess we're just trying to get on with living. We have to."

October 1996

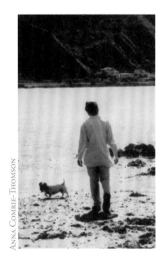

OPENING MY STUDIO DOOR, I notice it's partly overcast with a pale yellow sun trying to convince me that spring is almost here. Janet, who drops Wendy off, has stopped working and is now Wendy's full-time caregiver. Lisa is back at work but spends time in the evenings and weekends with her.

Wendy looks sad and tired this morning and her cough is troublesome. In spite of all these obstacles, she has still managed to bake muffins. We sit, savouring them and enjoying each other's company.

"All this must be quite hard for you."

She talks about her aching body, her cough, the constant reminders of her deteriorating health. Her sadness, almost despair, of leaving her family and the pain it will cause them. "Mum and I cry together. We manage to laugh as well. That feels good. And I write a lot in my diary."

"What else helps your sadness?"

"Spending time by myself, walking along the beach. I meditate often during the night. Sometimes I'm shown worlds of …" She searches for the right words, "… indescribable beauty. There I find the strength to carry my grief. I draw and write afterwards about my experiences."

She gives me her diary to read. The date is the 2nd of October.

The words have a beautiful simplicity and grace. "Thank you for letting me read this. This diary is a good companion."

"Yes," she agrees, "I can tell her anything. I'm still sorting out how I want my funeral, where I want my ashes and I'm writing a will. It'll still take some time but I want to finish it all in December."

I interrupt her. "Wendy, it's very thoughtful of you to organise all this for your family, but I still feel there's some living to do. You're concentrating a lot on your death and that's very courageous of you, but it still might take a while."

2 october

here i am
within my own little world tonight...
looking at things i can see my saying goodbye as steps ; steps
in which some parts of me physically begin to change or hurt and
steps in which the most important parts like my child and love
expand and reach upwards.
i know that it is okay for me to want to die . this thought in some
light makes me feel very sad but i still know it to be true
   while in another light it is perfectly comfortable and i'd be
happy to die tomorrow if i was too .
   sometimes and i know it is gaining on me , my body is not
pleasant to be within at all and i find it all so tiring .
   even if this body of mine feels pretty good , i find me being
sick , tiring . and again sometimes and i know it is
increasing are my glimpses of home . feelings of my angels and
guardian friends within a place of indescribable beauty where i
find comfort and pearls of love all around me

       and my sadness , my enormous sadness comes when i
   think of my family and angel friends here and
saying good bye to them for a while
                another step
                my love

She speaks with composure. "You know Mary Inglis, the hospital social worker who helped when I was diagnosed? I asked her to take me to some funeral homes. I wanted to meet the people there."

Wendy tells me how she and Mary visited several funeral homes. When it became obvious that Wendy was inquiring about her own funeral, the staff in some of the homes had difficulty handling it.

"I went ahead and chose a funeral director, a young woman. She didn't mind all my questions and I've made all the arrangements."

I sit listening, dumbfounded. Wendy notices and says with a slightly reassuring tone, "I know everything will work out. I really like her, she'll be good."

I eat another muffin and drink my herbal tea, hardly noticing that it's stone cold.

"Any drawings?"

"Yes, two more."

I see an angel or winged creature. "Is she around you as well?"

"Yes, sometimes. When I work with Raven she's always there."

Her next drawing is beautifully balanced, centred. A vibrant, radiating energy.

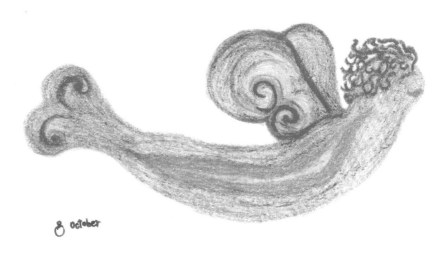

8 october

A butterfly still in gestation, waiting to birth again. I count sixteen petals, slowly opening into completion. It reminds me of a picture I have of the throat chakra.

"I have something here I want you to read." I go to my bookcase and take a folder from the shelf.

"These are some notes and illustrations I've collected over the years on chakras, our subtle energy centres."

I rummage through the many papers in my folder. "Here it is. This is the one." I give her the typed page.

"It's really a sort of summary of my own notes from different books."

Wendy reads it aloud:

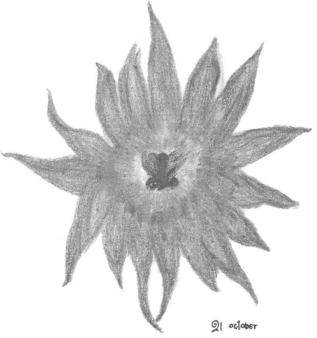

21 october

> In Eastern philosophies we find many writings and teachings on chakras or subtle energy centres of the body, each governing a different set of qualities and invisible to the eye.

> They lie like vortices or wheels along an inner pathway from the base of the spine to the top of the head. The major chakras all lie along this inner pathway. The chakras are often referred to as lotuses with varying numbers of petals. The fifth centre, at the region of the throat, is called the Visuddha chakra. Visuddha [Sanskrit] means 'pure'.

> It is said that when this centre is purified, we gain access to wisdom beyond human understanding. The Visuddha chakra is referred to as the gateway of great liberation. Great beings and sages tell us there is a beautiful, ethereal region, circular like the full moon, surrounded by sixteen petals, at the centre of this chakra."

Wendy repeats the words. " … 'wisdom beyond human understanding' … beyond the capacity of our mind to understand, to grasp it? Is that what it means, do you think?"

"Yes. Your insights around life and death, your connectedness with the beings you perceive around you during your meditation, your experiences of the different worlds that you visit with Raven, all those are not explainable by the human mind. And yes, we can read and study and come to intellectual explanations, but only if we ourselves are the perceiver or receiver of those experiences will we truly know. And that knowing is the awareness and integration of wisdom."

I feel pulled into the energy of the drawing in front of me.

Janet arrives and Wendy gets up. She gathers her things to leave and starts coughing again as she does so. "This always happens when I do anything remotely physical. Not a lot of transformation there."

"I'll make an appointment for you with the hospice, they might be able to help you with that cough."

I wave goodbye and walk back to the studio, contemplating once again the power of creativity. I am always intrigued by numerical symbolism. Wendy's drawings are spontaneous and she certainly is not consciously drawing sixteen petals.

November 1996

W HEN WENDY ARRIVES THIS MORNING she's accompanied by Lisa, who sits in on our session.

"How are you? Tired?"

"Yes, I have to rest in the afternoons now. I can't even go to the movies with Lisa any more. That means no hot chocolates with lots of marshmallows, eh Lise? Another piece the sculptor has chipped away." She smiles wryly. "I wonder what the next bit will be."

"Are you still writing everything down for your service and making all the arrangements?"

"Yes. I want a blue coffin with white clouds painted on it. I'll ask Reuben to do that."

"It will be a work of art, no doubt. You're still friends with Reuben?"

"Oh, yes, we'll always be friends." She changes the topic: "I've been quite busy actually, we're moving house in two weeks and I'm trying to pack some things."

"Are you looking forward to that?"

"Yes." She lights up at the thought. "My new room will have a beautiful view over Island Bay and the sea. I can watch the moon at night and see her reflection in the water."

She turns towards me. "Oh, I almost forgot. Do you think Anna would take some photos for me?"

Anna is a photographer and a good friend of mine.

"I want to use the photos as presents … for later."

We all three know what 'later' means.

"Sure, I'll ask her and she can call you to arrange something. Perhaps Raven can come as well, and the four of us can have a picnic somewhere."

Wendy beams. "I'd love that."

"Good. Your cough seems better. Do you still get short of breath?"

"Yes, but as long as I use my inhalers and pills and potions, it's really not too bad."

"You must tell Hetty about next Saturday," says Lisa.

"Oh, yes, next week Mum, Dad, Rachel, Lisa and I are going to Waimapihi Reserve in Aro Valley."

I give her a blank stare.

"I forgot to tell you. You know I want to be cremated and I've decided that half my ashes will go out to the sea, but I want the other half in a place where my family and others can visit. I found this reserve and I've got permission to plant an Astelia there. It's a New Zealand native and my ashes will be spread around it. So next Saturday we will all go with my plant and a picnic lunch."

"Right, a family picnic on Saturday in the reserve," I pronounce.

"We could have our other picnic with Anna and Raven there as well, and then you can all see my chosen spot."

"That sounds a good idea, I'd love to see the reserve and your Astelia."

I'm watching Lisa while Wendy is calmly talking about her plans, her ashes, her picnics and her blue 'white-clouded' coffin. It's obvious that Lisa's doing her utmost not to cry and make it difficult for Wendy.

"This must be tough for you, listening to all this, Lisa?"

Lisa shrugs, unable to talk. She blows her nose and her eyes are full of tears. Wendy stands and gives her a hug.

"I love you, Lisa," she says softly.

As they leave I hear Lisa suggesting that they stop somewhere for a hot chocolate and lots of marshmallows.

I reflect on Wendy. The many tears she's shed, her terror and fears she faced so courageously. Her work with Raven. The endless nights sitting by herself trying to accept the inevitable and facing the unknown ahead of her. It's paid off, and now she's able to sit here and calmly talk about preparations for the funeral and her own death.

As planned, the family all go on Saturday to the reserve and plant the little native, the 'Silver Spear'. It is the creation of a special place. Lisa later tells me, "It was a magical, surreal day — we cried and we laughed. The sun was shining and birds were singing and Mum brought a picnic lunch and everyone agreed it was an enjoyable day!"

I ask Lisa how she copes with Wendy's deteriorating health.

"It is really, really hard. I keep asking myself if there's a right way to act. I read books to try and find answers, but there's nothing that helps you determine whether what you're doing is right. I long for a sense of normality, but nothing's normal any more. I have so much love to give Wendy, but I feel guilty if I spend time with other people. I have a boyfriend now, James. I feel guilty if I spend time with him, yet I need to, to get strength to support and comfort her. And if I don't spend time with him, I almost feel resentful and that makes me feel guilty again. It's a strange guilt, not having enough time to give everyone their share of me."

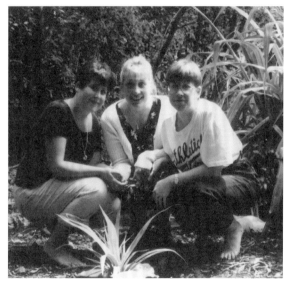

Wendy, Lisa and Rachel with the Astelia.

"It's amazing how guilt always manages to get us, no matter what we do. Nobody can tell you how to be, what to do. Always be honest, tell Wendy, tell James how you feel. You don't have to keep it all inside."

"I have my diary. Almost every day I write how I feel and what's happening. Sometimes that helps me make sense of it all. I go to acting and drama classes, that's what I really love to do. I can let it all out."

"What about your new job?"

"I'm lacking any motivation. I'm at work, but my mind's somewhere else completely, thinking about Wendy, thinking about how I'll get through today and tomorrow and next week. I can hardly think about what's ahead of us. The unknown is really the hardest. I know that when her life has finished, our lives without Wendy in this world will begin. And I really don't want to think about it, it's too awful.

"Wendy was so sad yesterday and yet she's organising her funeral, down to the last detail. You know how thorough our Wenz is. I feel so alone at times, it feels like she's already moving away from me." *

* Lisa Potter from 'Many Rivers to Cross'

Later that month Wendy, Raven, Anna and I have our day out. Numerous photos are taken on the beach, in the reserve and with and without Wendy's dog, Jessie.

Wendy makes an incredible effort and although tired, she manages to be very photogenic and demonstrates a healthy appetite for the French bread and cheeses, and a dessert of Dutch chocolate. While Anna and Wendy are taking photos around the plant, Raven and I decide to walk through the reserve. A fantail follows us, making sure we hear its chatter.

Anna, Raven, Wendy and Hetty.

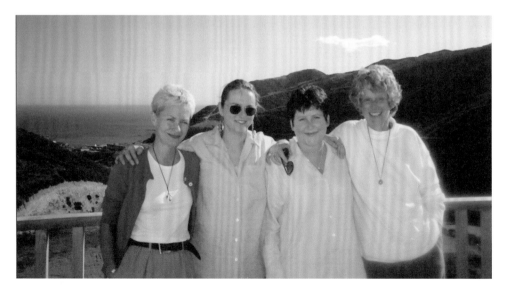

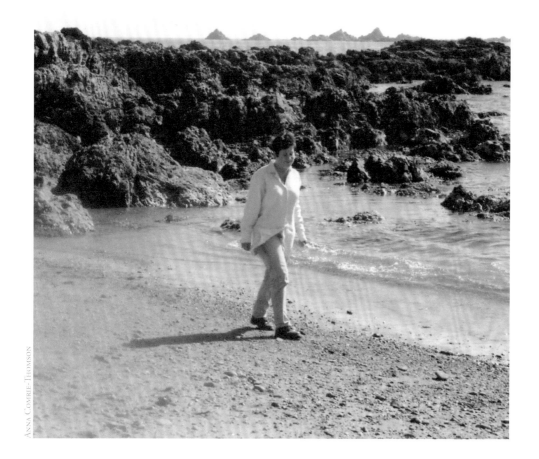

December 1996

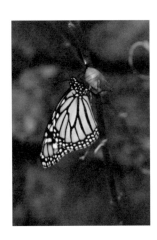

"WHAT ARE YOU DOING FOR CHRISTMAS?"
"Christmas is different for me this year, I don't want any presents."
"Oh? When did you make that decision?"

"I've been thinking about it for a while. I know this is my last Christmas. I don't need anything and I have gifts for my family and friends when I die. That's important for me. I told my family last night."

"Wendy, have you considered that they might want to give you something? If you don't allow that, you take away the gift of giving."

"They give me love, Hetty, in so many ways, that's their gift. That's what I receive daily."

"That's very true and I accept your feeling that time is running out, yet their need might be to celebrate Christmas as normally as possible."

"Yes." She seems to be lost in thought. "You're probably right. Mum and Dad are sad. I know Mum will do anything I ask of her, but Lisa got quite upset. We had a talk later."

Wendy talks once again about her feeling that she's going to die around Christmas.

"I have to say this again, you seem to be waiting for death to arrive, you have even set a time. Remember, when our soul decides to be free again, then we die. Not a moment before or after. It's like the caterpillar, the cocoon and the butterfly. Metamorphosis is taking place inside and the butterfly appears at the perfect time."

Wendy is listening attentively, but I have a strong feeling she is sticking to her own agenda. "Well, here is my butterfly," she says, tongue in cheek. I smile at her.

She pushes her drawing book in front of me and I study the picture.

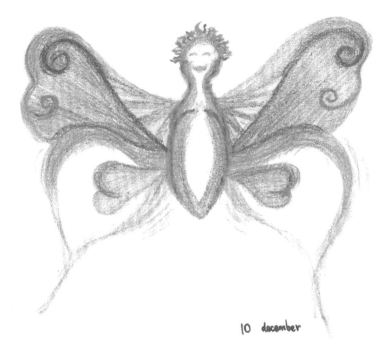

10 december

Quite a cheery butterfly with a happy smile. The lower wings look fragile to me. Are they strong enough for flying? Is this butterfly ready to be released from the restrictions of the cocoon?

"Tell me about your drawing."

"I have a sense of completion." She touches the paper. "That moment in time, the end of my journey, feels not too far away."

I wonder if this is really Wendy's last drawing.

After Wendy has left, I sit in the sun, listening to the birds. I start to doubt my own thoughts and feelings about Wendy's time of death. Do I need to change my Christmas holiday plans? I will discuss it with my partner tonight.

Wendy phones. She's forgotten her scarf, so the next day, when I'm in town for a meeting, I drop it off. Janet is home alone. Lisa and Wendy have gone to the reserve to see how the little plant is doing. I admire the new house, the open-plan kitchen, the dining room and lounge. There's a beautiful view over the sea and hills of Island Bay and the sun is streaming in, lighting the white, painted walls. We have coffee and talk.

"I just go on, minute by minute, day to day, what else can I do? Ever since my children were born, if anyone had asked me what my worst nightmare was, it would've been that something had happened to my children. I remember the overwhelming feeling I had when Wendy was diagnosed with cancer. The feeling that this can't be happening to us, and at the same time trying to face up to it and help Wendy in whatever way I could."

She puts her yellow coffee mug down. "I still try to keep a sense of normality. Life continues. Cyril and Lisa go to work, come home, we have dinner, we go to sleep. And then there's my father. He needs time, especially since Mum died. He doesn't say much, but I know he's devastated with what's happening to Wendy. And there's always washing, cooking, shopping; in a small way the routine keeps me sane.

"Wendy keeps talking about dying and she's preparing herself and us with so much love and precision, but it's all so unreal. Like I said before, it's my worst nightmare coming true. There are times when I cry and want to scream that it's so unfair. Sometimes when I'm by myself, I do scream and it helps a little. Every day something dies. Wendy told us the other night about no Christmas presents this year. Did she mention that when she saw you?"

"Yes, she did. I questioned her motivations. How do you feel about it?"

"Sad. I think Lisa's quite angry. It's another reminder that this Christmas and all other Christmases will never be the same."

"How is Cyril?"

Janet hesitates. "He works hard and sometimes goes away on the weekends, four-wheel driving. I think it helps him, and yet at the same time it's a reminder that Wendy's not with him. We don't have a lot of communication, he's so angry and resentful that all this is happening to him and his family, to his daughter. He says it's like living in hell. Well, he isn't the only one. We're all living in our own hell."

We finish our coffee. Janet sighs, then turns to me. "Oh, I must tell you what happened the other day. Wendy wanted to do some shopping and we went to some dress shops in Willis Street. We were both looking through the racks of dresses when she suddenly announced she was really wanting something to wear for her funeral.

"I stood in the shop with my mouth open, trying not to burst into tears. In the end she chose a greeny-blue dress and said, 'This is the one I'll wear, just once'."

I'm not sure if I want to cry or laugh, hearing Janet's story.

One of Janet's friends arrives and I go upstairs to Wendy's room to deposit the forgotten scarf. On her bed are numerous stones, shells and leaves. I know Wendy will paint them in vibrant colours, perhaps write some words, little messages of her love. There are quite a few framed photographs with a personal message from Wendy written on them, waiting to be carefully wrapped. A bed covered with love.

For a few minutes I stand there, very still. I hang Wendy's scarf over Bessie, her big white teddy bear.

January 1997

CHRISTMAS HAS BEEN AND GONE, and I offer to see Wendy at home, hoping it will give me a chance to talk to other family members as well. Janet is home when I arrive, Cyril and Lisa are still at work, and Wendy is resting in her room upstairs. Janet and I have a coffee together and she tells me how hard it is for everybody.

"I'll never forget this Christmas. Wendy wrote the final preparations for her funeral and wrapped all the presents she's made for us, to be given after her death. She told me she'd finished everything. She really expected to die around Christmas. I went shopping and bought small presents for everybody. On Christmas Day my dad came over and Wendy made a huge effort to stay up, and even managed to eat something. So here we were with our Christmas tree and candles and all of us trying to behave naturally, and yet all of us thinking about it and not knowing if it would happen."

"It must have been such a difficult time. For quite a while I've been concerned with Wendy's preoccupation with her death. It's common for patients at this stage in their illness to have a need to get ready, to finish things, to have precious time with family and friends and to create a sense of completion. But it's been slightly different with Wendy. Her insistence on her time of dying made it quite confusing for me as well."

"Yes. We all believed her and perhaps psyched ourselves up for that moment. It was so frightening."

I notice how tired Janet looks.

"I hope you get out now and then, go for a meal, have a talk with your friends, have some walks along the beach. You need breaks, otherwise you'll burn out. Try to share more as a family. I don't know how long all this is going to last."

"Sometimes you do want to know and then you don't. All at the same time."

"Yes. And perhaps thankfully, that answer belongs to the universe or to God.

Perhaps Wendy's realised this, and by allowing herself to relax a little it gives her body some breathing space, metaphorically speaking."

"Perhaps that's what's happening in Wendy's body. At the moment she almost seems to have a little more energy and she's eating slightly better."

We are both silent. Jessie, Wendy's dog, snores loudly in the sun.

Janet's face lights up. "I need to tell you something, you'll love this. I sleep quite badly, always anxious that Wendy might need me. Sometimes I wonder what I'll see when I bring her a cup of a tea in the morning. A few nights ago when I'd been asleep a few hours, I suddenly woke up and the room was lit up with this beautiful white shimmering light. I sat up and for a moment I wasn't sure if it was a dream. I felt this indescribable presence of love and peace. I got up to see Wendy, wondering if something had happened, but when I opened her door she just looked at me and said: 'It's all right, Mum, I'm still here'.

"That feeling stayed with me for quite a time. It's the most beautiful present I've ever received. I know now I'll have the strength to go through this, I'll never be alone."

I go upstairs to see Wendy. She opens her eyes when I enter her bedroom. "I heard you talking with Mum."

I hug her. "Well, here we are. Not such a 'Happy New Year,' is it?"

"No, it's not. I'm not dead but I don't feel alive either. Suspended between two worlds. In my dreams and meditations I'm at peace. I have a feeling of just being. Now. Here. But I can't hold that feeling when I wake up. My body hurts and I'm tired, and I feel I've had enough of it."

"Perhaps, and it might be quite difficult for you, perhaps you need to surrender into that here and now. Be in it. Remember the aeroplane and the pilot seat?"

"Yes and I guess I'm still sitting on one wing."

"That's right, you're a little out of balance. You need to get back into that pilot seat, in the centre and accept both wings again."

"I don't feel like flying, I feel like landing."

"You haven't been given the okay from the tower yet."

Wendy's eyes close and after a few minutes she nods off. I tiptoe from the room.

February 1997

IT'S GOING TO BE A GORGEOUS DAY, and I get up early to have a walk and a swim in the sea. I love the beach, and seeing the first rays of light appearing over the hill. There are two other swimmers and we are in total agreement about the sustenance this early exercise affords.

Wendy arrives after nine. "I like being here with you in this beautiful studio, the trees and the birds outside, your garden full of flowers."

We drink our tea and eat our muffins, and for a few minutes life is just an appreciation of the senses. My dog Harvey, who always likes to be present when Wendy's here, nudges her gently.

"Oh, I almost forgot you." She gives Harvey a huge pat.

"I've something for you. I wrote it the other night." Wendy hands me a small piece of paper.

to hetty with love

being within your company
is like sitting upon stars of divinity
or standing in the shade
of a wise old tree
or lieing within a field
of wild daisies

when im sad you're comforting
like a love fairy
your smile warms my heart
and makes me happy
my friend the love between us
will always be
for it is like a flower
forever blossoming free
i love you
Wendy

"Thank you, this is very special."

"That's how I feel."

I feel moved by her beautiful words and give her a big hug.

Finally I ask, "How are you? How are things?"

"Not much has changed. I feel tired, sleep a lot, try to eat to please Mum … try very hard to embrace both wings of my aeroplane, but I find it such an effort. There are times I don't want to be here. I want it over and done with. And when I think it might take months I feel so sad. I just go back to sleep again."

I wonder if Wendy is depressed. "This is very hard for you. Even though you are tired and have lost a lot of weight, your body's still the body of a 19 year old. It's strong and it's not giving up easily. You've been given astonishing understanding, insights and visions in your dreams and meditations, which perhaps make it all the more appealing to leave and harder to stay. But living until we die is a process which has its own timing."

"Here's your 'surrender' again, that you talked about last time."

"Yes, letting yourself just 'be'. Like floating down a river that will bring you to the ocean."

"That sounds nice. I'm too tired to swim any more."

"As long as you keep your head above the water, you might even enjoy the scenery."

"A sight to behold."

"Remember we talked about still having choices? You can choose how you want to be, even if that's the most difficult thing you still have to do."

"Sometimes it's hard to remember that I still have choices."

"Yes, and not easy when you're so tired. It might help you if you can find some more structure in your life: small outings, a drive in the car and going somewhere for a cup of hot chocolate if you feel up to that. Watch a video, sit in the garden, draw something, write. You have friends. There's still much to exchange, to enjoy with each other. In times like this, the small things in life mean the most."

"Thank you, I will really try."

A moment later Lisa's car pulls into the driveway.

"Wenz, I won't be a moment, just want to ask Hetty something. Sit in the car if you like, it's nice and warm with the sun shining into it." We both watch as Wendy climbs into the car, makes herself comfortable in the front seat, and closes her eyes.

"She'll be asleep in a minute. Sometimes I feel scared to enjoy Wendy, and I think, do I just need to keep preparing myself for her death? And how do you keep preparing yourself for loss?"

I put my arm around her shoulders. "Perhaps the answer is life itself … is in living. Enjoy Wendy and the outings and time you spend together. Talk like you have always talked. Laugh with her, cry with her. Never be afraid to show your love. Never be afraid to show your grief. Be present with her. Now."

"I guess in Western societies we're not very prepared for grief or mourning."

"No. And it's not part of our culture, which is so devoid of rituals, so it doesn't make it any easier. Our Western society moved away from the sacredness of death, and grief and ritual, a long time ago. But, no matter what time and culture we live in we can never prepare ourselves for the experience of the loss, that unbearable pain. Ask for help when you need it. Get away, use nature as a nurturer."

We walk towards the car. Wendy is fast asleep, her head in the sun.

"Nature is looking after her," says Lisa with a smile.

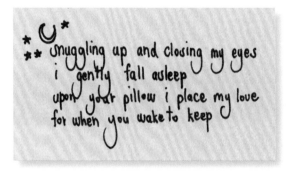

snuggling up and closing my eyes
i gently fall asleep
upon your pillow i place my love
for when you wake to keep

Studio 2005

I'M BACK FROM A WALK through the bush behind my house and a coffee in my favourite café on the waterside, and I feel energised.

I'm ready to write about April 1997. First I read the letters from the hospice, then my own notes:

> Start of severe abdominal pain, primarily in the morning. Cough causing her to be very quickly short of breath. Decision made to start her on a subcutaneous morphine pump for symptom management. Only partial improvement.
> Suggest admission to hospice for pain control.

I visited Wendy during that time and watched Janet caring for her daughter, rubbing her back, wiping Wendy's forehead when she was in pain. I remember so vividly their deep affection and respect for one another.

Janet's life had come to revolve solely around Wendy. The last dance, with Janet aware and aligned to every move Wendy made.

April 1997

I RECEIVE A LETTER from the hospice and am thankful for Rod MacLeod's input. He's extremely skilful in addressing the difficulties associated with the 'prolonged dying' phase.

15 April 1997

re: Wendy Potter; d.o.b. 7.7.77

It was a pleasure to see Wendy again following her discharge from the hospice. During that time we had been able to alleviate her intermittent abdominal pain and she went home having felt that the visit to the hospice was very successful.

On this occasion I talked with her at some length about the difficulties associated with the 'prolonged dying' phase. I talked of the necessity for us to try and help her to concentrate on living, rather than focus on the dying, and during that discussion it transpired that Wendy still sees some days as being very black and bleak and she feels that she is unable to get out of bed because 'there is no point'. I was trying to work out in my own mind whether or not she was clinically depressed but at present I am really uncertain. I talked with her about linking with Linda, our occupational therapist, who has done some very useful and productive art work and I am hopeful that we may be able to persuade Wendy to come to the Day Unit to follow that medium.

I would very much like to see Wendy again and have given her an appointment for a month. If you have a chance I would be interested to talk with you on the telephone about just where we are.

On a purely medical note she commented that she is having more night sweats. These could be alleviated by a small dose of Thioridazine, say 10mgs taken at night. She could probably reduce the Haloperidol now as well.

Now that Wendy is back home again, I decide to visit her to see if there are any changes in her sometimes bleak outlook. Janet and I have our usual coffee and talk about the view and the weather, and for a few minutes we can almost create a reality where Wendy and cancer are just onlookers.

"Cyril's been offered counselling in the hospice. I'm glad he's accepted the idea of seeing someone."

"Yes, the hospice counsellors are fantastic, and they will know Wendy as well."

"I'm so glad Wendy's pain is much better controlled now with the new drugs. She's attending the hospice's Day Unit for art therapy once or twice a week and seems to have thrown herself into the art of silk painting with great enthusiasm. It's definitely helping her focus more on day-to-day living. We all feel a sense of relief, knowing that she's not so down any more." Janet gets up and shows me Wendy's latest product.

"What stunning colours, this should be framed and …"

"… preserved for future generations? It certainly will be."

A familiar voice makes me turn around. Wendy stands in the doorway, fully dressed. I look at her in awe. Yet another one of Wendy's surprising metamorphoses has taken place. She's vibrant in a brightly coloured shirt and jeans, and a recent new rinse through her hair.

"Close your mouth, I'm going out for lunch with Mum. I've got some living to do."

I pick up my car keys from the table. "Wendy, you're a star. Have a great lunch."

A few days later I receive a phone call from Janet. "Thought you'd like to hear this, Wendy's gone on a shopping spree and bought new clothes. What do you think of that?"

I laugh. "I'm trying hard not to think, Janet. After all, this is Wendy. I'm getting used to her all-or-nothing approach. I must admit the 'all' is easier to work with."

Next Saturday, during the intermission of a concert, I bump into Rachel. We talk about Wendy, and Rachel mentions her feelings of inadequacy when she visits her family.

"I want to see Wendy, but it seems that everybody has a role in caring for her. I don't feel a part of that any more."

"Yes, I can understand that, Rachel. Does Chris come with you?"

"No," Rachel admits, slightly uncomfortable. "Chris and Dad had an argument and Chris refuses to visit my family now. He's my husband and I have chosen to support him. Of course I want to see Wendy, she's my sister. Lisa made a remark the other day as well, that I really should come and see Wendy a little more often.

"I'll try to go tomorrow. Nobody knows how long Wendy has with us."

The sound of the bell brings us to a different reality and we walk back to the hall.

May 1997

WENDY HOLDS UP a beautiful painted silk butterfly. "For your collection. Now you can have a silk one as well."

"It's a work of art, destined to brighten my days." I carefully hang it over a chair. "Do you like the art classes?"

"Very much, and it's good to get out of the house. It's fun and the staff are inspiring. I feel whole when I'm creative and …" Wendy grins at me, "my cancer is definitely not driving my bus when I'm in the hospice Day Unit."

"Are you tired afterwards?"

"Exhausted is a better word, but I guess it's all worth it."

"Life seems a little brighter for you."

"Yes. I enjoy my little outings. I only had one shopping spree, by the way. My family exaggerates this occasion. I love to go out and watch the trees slowly losing their leaves for winter. Or to smell the sea on a windy day.

"I feel the family changing. Mum and Dad don't talk a lot with each other, Rachel comes to visit but not very often. And Lisa tries to find time for both James and for me and is stressed to the max."

"You're not responsible for the way people respond to your illness. It affects many people and they all move around you and each other like different pieces on the chessboard of life. But how they move, how they communicate is their choice and their responsibility."

"I know that, I just want to help them and I feel so powerless."

"Perhaps it's not your task to help them. Your love's holding your family together and will always support them in their sadness and feelings of loss. Their challenge is how to remain true to their feelings for you and each other and, at the same time, find the right time and place to express those feelings. And this drama plays against the backdrop of what existed before you became ill: the relationships that were already challenged. I'm talking about the emotional battlefields that can happen in any family."

"Is my family dying as well?"

"Your family are dealing with a huge transformation — and I want you to know that you are not responsible."

"I do know that. I just wish I could make it all better." She leaves soon after.

Standing in front of the open window, I hold my new silk gift up towards the light. The fabric moves in the wind and the spotted wings of my new butterfly seem almost to flutter.

I receive a phone call from Lisa.

"Wendy wants to go overseas to Noosa, in Australia, where it's warm. She wants me to go with her."

For a moment I'm speechless. "How do you feel about that?"

"How do I feel about that? In one word, not bloody good. I love Wendy to bits and would do anything for her, but not Noosa. There are limits to my confidence. She's just not strong enough. What if something happens?"

"Have you talked about that?"

"I'm just waiting and hoping she'll change her mind. If she really insists, we'll need to renegotiate and find a warm place in New Zealand."

"Could be a bit of a challenge in the winter," I say lightly.

"Yeah, but nothing like the Noosa challenge."

We both laugh and agree.

"Anyway, I just wanted to let you know in case Wendy calls you."

"Thanks. With Wendy's determination I might see you at the airport."

"I don't think so."

June 1997

WENDY NEEDS PRESCRIPTIONS and makes a flying visit to the surgery while Janet waits outside in the car.

"Where did you end up going for the holiday?"

"Taupo, Napier and in between. Wasn't necessarily warm, but just having the week with Lisa was worth it. And to indulge in hot chocolates and ice creams again. Mind you, my ability to keep things down has become unpredictable. But at least I had a taste of everything. Including freedom."

"You make it all sound like fun. I'm sure it wasn't all that easy."

"True, I felt awful for Lisa when I was sick again. But we managed to find something funny in everything. It helps when you have a slightly warped sense of humour. It's helped me through many embarrassing moments."

"What did you do during the day?"

"The agenda was carefully built around my siestas. But we did Marineland, the occasional movie and cafés." She becomes serious. "This was the last time for Lisa and me and I can't tell you how much it's meant to me."

I walk her out to the car to say hello to Janet. "I hope you lived dangerously while your daughters were away!"

She laughs. "They were back on the doorstep before I had energy to even think about it. Now I'm reading *Chicken Soup for the Soul* to Wendy. It's the third time — she tends to fall asleep halfway through."

"That's my mum. She's the best."

Lisa tells me later, "It was wonderful to spend time with Wendy, to have this adventure with her. Worth everything, even the times that I had to carry our stuff up and down to the car and look after Wendy at the same time. We laughed lots, the food was good, the weather surprisingly wonderful and the sunsets gorgeous."

"Was it more difficult than you'd imagined?"

"Yes, it was emotionally challenging. I was devastated when Wendy was sick, I felt so helpless during the frequent bouts of vomiting. I was frightened at night when I heard her laboured breathing, stopping and starting. Sometimes I wanted to scream: breathe, breathe!"

"And did you scream?"

"No, I prayed."

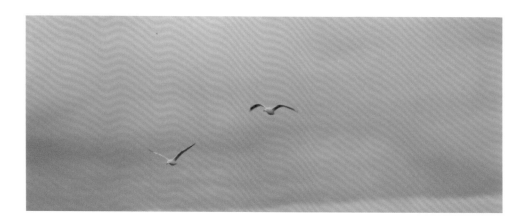

Studio 2005

I READ OVER MY NOTES from the last part of 1997.

Wendy sleeps more, eats less.
Frequent bouts of vomiting.
Pain is reasonably controlled. Uses
morphine elixir for breakthrough pain.
Regular visits of district nurses.
Rae Elliot, charge district nurse, great
help and support to family.

July 1997

I RING HER. "Happy birthday! I hope you'll have a great day."

She sounds pleased. "I'll call you tomorrow and tell you all about it. If I can remember any of it, that is."

I imagine how difficult this day will be for Wendy's family. The fact that nobody expected Wendy to be still alive beyond last Christmas must create emotional havoc at times. The certainty of knowing her death is imminent, yet at the same time the sense of gratitude that she's still here. It challenges the mind to make sense of it all.

As Lisa once said: "There are moments when I wonder whether I dare to feel the joy her presence creates. We live with the day-to-day existence of not knowing, and simultaneously there's the dreaded knowing that it is going to happen."

The next day when Wendy calls, she is exhausted.

"It was great, but I'm so tired. Lots of flowers and phone calls. I slept a lot, but when my granddad came I managed to stay awake and talk with him. We went to my favourite Indian restaurant."

I'm sure I must have misheard her. "An Indian restaurant?"

"Yeah, you should've seen Mum and Dad's face when I suggested it. I knew you'd be surprised, and not only did I get dressed, I ate a decent amount and didn't fall asleep during the dinner. My family was on tenterhooks, but I managed to behave until I came home, then I lost my favourite curry in the now familiar way. Worth it though, it was a great evening."

"You certainly don't allow your cancer to limit your culinary choices, do you?"

"Well, you've always told me there is only the now. So as long as there are still nows, I'd better use them. You see how good a student I am?"

"You're a good teacher as well, Wendy. You always give me some food for thought."

"If I were you, I'd just stick to the thought."

Studio 2005

I REMEMBER WENDY'S BIRTHDAY as one of the last bursts of energy. It was short-lived and her condition then took a turn for the worse.

Notes:

Phone call from Rae: Wendy is vomiting and exhausted.
Difficulty walking to bathroom and going downstairs
to living room.
Food intake quite low. Drinks fluids.
Appears to be vague and distant. Change medication.
Phone call from Rae two days later: No improvement.
Admit to hospice for symptom control.

Late July 1997

WHEN I WALK INTO WENDY'S ROOM at the hospice I'm amazed to find her quite rosy, chatting away with Lisa and greeting me with open arms. My surprise must be obvious.

"You doctors aren't used to miracles!"

"And how was this miracle engineered?"

"Easily. Two blood transfusions and new wonder drugs." She taps the little bag which holds the syringe driver. "I'm getting them through this subcutaneous syringe driver, or as the nurses call it, the pump."

She spreads out her arms. "*Et voilà*, a new Wendy."

I wonder if the 'new Wendy' could be a little high on her morphine. She certainly seems ready to continue the battle.

"Raven's coming too. She called this morning and asked if I was allowed visitors."

Raven laughingly calls me a day later. "Would you like to hear a story about rabbits, Wendy and morphine?"

"Enlighten me. This does not create an instant medical reference for me."

"Well, you know I see Wendy every week. She's been to our house and fallen in love with our menagerie, especially the rabbit, who's now the proud mother of two little ones. I knew Wendy was in the hospice, so yesterday the three of us went to visit."

"The three of you?"

"Yes, my learned friend. Me and the two four-legged fluffy ones. They travel well in a handbag. Anyway, Wendy was beside herself, they were all over her bed and face and chest. She absolutely loved them. And there was this nurse who was equally entranced. Shows you they don't see enough rabbits there! Anyway I noticed one of the little ones was behaving oddly and kept falling over on Wendy's chest. After a closer look we discovered she'd made a little hole in the tube connecting the needle with the pump, and had taken little sips of morphine, which went down very well. The nurse was fantastic, she was laughing just as much as we were. She very obligingly got a nice new tube for Wendy's pump and the little darlings went back in their travel bag. Apparently the nurses hung the gnawed tube on the noticeboard for a few days, with the warning: 'Beware, rabbits should not be allowed to chew the equipment'."

A few days later I received a discharge letter from the hospice.

Date of admission:	21.7.97	Wendy Potter; d.o.b. 7.7.77;
Date of discharge:	25.7.97	
Diagnosis:		Stage IV Hodgkin's Lymphoma

Wendy was admitted to our care through the night on 20 July with nausea, vomiting and difficulty managing her oral medications. Her family were exhausted and Wendy also was complaining of shortness of breath and extreme tiredness.

Wendy was commenced on a subcutaneous driver syringe containing Morphine 300mgs, Cyclizine 150mgs and Maxolon 40mgs all over 24 hours. On this regime her nausea and vomiting quickly settled. Her haemoglobin was found to be low, at 86grams/litre so she was transfused 2 units of packed cells on 22 July, with benefit. Her haemoglobin thereafter rose to 111 grams/litre.

By 25 July she was keen to be discharged home and a symptom control appointment has been arranged for approximately two weeks time. Rae Elliott will continue to be closely involved, as I am sure you will yourself.

During Wendy's admission her mother Janet spent considerable time with one of our counsellors, who will continue to support her now that Wendy is at home. We would of course be happy to re-admit Wendy at any time, should you feel this necessary.

26 July

here i am
inside my bedroom, full of warmth and love while
outside the wind never slows down and the rain
continues to fall
i am safe
i think of my Nana
of a very special spirit who is forever around
me and always in my heart
i love her so and welcome her embrace
tonight I thought of how I no longer want any
battles. i want my hurt to be free so i no
longer carry it upon me and I know my
luggage of sadness is bearing lighter
for i want to be me, i want to
be light so i can shine

August 1997

WENDY IS FAST ASLEEP on the couch in the living room. I sit next to her, watching her for a while. A table near the wall is covered with reminders of Wendy's cancer. Her medical charts, her medication in different coloured boxes with pharmaceutical names on them, a little tray with bandages and sterile swabs, ampoules for the pump, saliva sticks, rubber gloves and the nurse's notebooks and diaries, daily recordings of Wendy's mortality.

I read through the last notes and check the drug charts.

"They might not have mentioned Wendy's dining-out adventure," Janet says with love and humour in her voice. "She wanted to go to Theatre Sports the other night and have dinner first."

"I don't believe it."

"Well, I can tell you we all reacted with a stunned silence, but she insisted. So we went to a Greek restaurant, Wendy's choice, followed by one-and-a-half hours of entertainment."

"And did she manage to stay awake?"

"Through the dinner yes, but she slept peacefully throughout most of the improvisation. When I helped her into bed she said: 'What a wonderful evening, I loved the acting'."

"Does she still surprise you?"

"Not so much what she does but how she does it. Yes, that still surprises me."

Wendy wakes. "Hi Hetty, I heard you talking with Mum."

"Did we disturb you?"

"You can always disturb me, I love to see you. How are you? Are you busy?"

"I'm fine, thanks."

"You look tired. You need to take care of yourself."

"Yes," I murmur, half amused and half chastened.

We enjoy each other's company. She has a few questions about the dose of her morphine and the pain in her legs. Before I leave she asks, "How long is it going to last?"

"I don't know, not too much longer hopefully. I can only assure you that we'll do everything we can to keep you comfortable."

"Raven was here yesterday and she gave me some healing. I had such a good sleep afterwards. She said the same as you when I asked her."

After a few moments, "I hope it won't be long."

Cyril arrives just as I'm getting into my car. We talk outside the house.

"How are you, Cyril?"

"Oh ... you know, couldn't be worse. And ..." his voice is slightly raised, "I'm just so angry with everything: the world, God, the doctors, myself."

"Why are you angry with yourself?"

"Sometimes I feel I'm responsible for her. I brought Wendy into this world and I feel responsible for all that pain she's going through. I wish I could die instead of her."

I give him a hug. No words will be enough, but I hope love and time will do their work.

September 1997

WHEN I ARRIVE, I notice quite a change in Wendy's physical appearance. She's frail, has obviously lost more weight and her eyes are slightly sunken.

I read the notes written by the visiting district nurses:

> Wendy sleeps most days. Very tired but appears to be peaceful.
> Cooperative, asks questions about medication.
> Refuses bedpan or commode.
> Vomiting ++. Increase fluid intake.

I sit on Wendy's bed, holding her hand. "I'm so tired. I don't know how long I can go on."

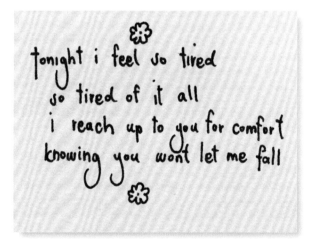

"I know … it won't be long."

"I'm ready to go, I know my angels will guide me, I'll never be alone. But … when is that going to happen?"

I don't answer. She closes her eyes. A few minutes later she implores, "Will you look after my family?"

"I will. I'll try to be there when they need me."

"Thank you."

"Will you talk at my funeral?"
"I will. Thank you for asking me. Is everything arranged?"

"I did everything last November, but I knew I could ask you at any time."

"You can ask me anything, any time."

She squeezes my hand and smiles.

"Who plays Monopoly?" I pick up the box from under a little side table.

"We play in the evenings with Wendy," Janet say. "She's developed a passion for it. You'd be surprised how she's able to concentrate on the game. We all sit around the coffee table and Wendy 'monopolises' the game from the couch. She cracks little jokes and wins most of the time."

I'm thoroughly amused by the image of Wendy buying and selling Pall Mall and the like, the shrewd businesswoman coming alive in the evenings.

"I know," Janet laughs. "It's such a special time and we all happily accept her superiority in the property market."

"Are you still able to take care of her by yourself? She needs so much more nursing care now."

"Sometimes it's not easy." Janet has made tea, and holding her cup in both hands, sits down and closes her eyes. Wendy coughs, and she immediately gets up and walks to the couch where Wendy is fast asleep. Janet pulls the blanket around her shoulders and gently strokes her face. A mother's love and a mother's grief are all in that one small gesture.

I pour us another cup of tea and Janet resumes. "The nurses are fantastic. I can call them any time. Yesterday I got such a fright. Wendy vomited so much and fainted in my arms. It was terrible. I thought she was going to die. Luckily one of the district nurses just arrived. They're coming three times a day now. They think Wendy has moved into the next stage."

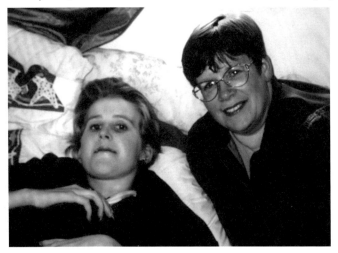

Wendy and Janet.

"I agree. We need to keep a good eye on her medication. Her morphine might need to be increased when her pain gets worse."

"Getting her out of bed to the toilet is a nightmare. We give her some morphine elixir before moving and lifting her. It's so excruciatingly painful for her. Her body's so thin and she bruises so easily."

"Have you suggested the commode again?"

"We all have, many times. She absolutely refuses. She's always had a will of her own, and I'm afraid the decision's been made, come what may. It's the same iron will which gets her to the toilet and back to bed. Wendy has never allowed her illness to run her life, so a commode's certainly not going to change that."

We both start to laugh.

"It's just as well we can laugh and cry at the same time."

"How is Wendy with the district nurses and the daily visits and care?"

"She never complains. Her approach to all the daily challenges is a mixture of determination, stubbornness, and humour. The other day Rae told me some of the things Wendy said about commodes, obviously in a state of some morphine euphoria. It was hilarious."

"There are only a few things left Wendy can say no to."

"Yes, and I'll do anything to make it easier for her."

After I arrive home friends come around for dinner. They comment that I am unusually quiet. I enjoy my glass of pinot gris and reflect on the tenacity of the human species.

October 1997

DISTRICT NURSES VISIT WENDY two to three times a day, spending more and more time with her. They adjust her medication regularly and help with the daily wash/sponge/toilet routine. A gentle touch to her painful and aching body.

During one of my visits I talk to Lisa, who has stopped working to share Wendy's full-time care with Janet.

Lisa is drained. "I feel so upset seeing Wendy existing like this, yet at the same time I've experienced some truly precious moments. Even though she sleeps a lot, she still has amazingly lucid periods and often makes astute comments and says the most fascinating things. I'm so grateful to be a part of it. Yesterday she wanted Mum and me to sort through her clothes to decide which ones would go charity and which ones Rachel and I might like. I carefully chose the clothes I'd love to have, either for sentimental reasons, or as reminders of special times or colours we both love. After I'd been through them, Wendy was very interested in knowing my choices and as I held up each article she nodded and said things like 'Yep, I knew you'd want that'. And she was quite adamant that the clothes were not to be worn or taken to a charity until after her death. She's still making the decisions here." *

* Lisa Potter
'Many Rivers to Cross'

Reuben is coming to visit. They haven't seen each other for a long time. Wendy insists on being dressed and chooses her clothes. "Can you do my hair and make-up, Lisa? And I want to sit in the wheelchair."

Janet and Lisa are busy following Wendy's instructions. When Reuben walks in, Wendy manages to stand and like old lovers they embrace. They hold hands and talk. Reuben has no problems understanding Wendy, even while her speech is often slurred and the contents of it are occasionally 'way out,' due to a combination of excitement and medication.

After Reuben has left, Wendy is utterly exhausted. Her last words before she falls asleep with a smile on her face are, "Reuben and I had a magical time."

I visit often. I'm just there, sharing thoughts, holding her hand, having cups of tea with the family. One afternoon she remarks, "Well, it's good that I did all my preparations last year, I couldn't have written a thing now."

I agree. "That's what you call completion."

"My suitcase is almost empty. I will travel very lightly."

"Yes, with a suitcase full of love. It'll be all around you like a cloak and it will hold you safely."

"That's how it feels, it's just this body that's the problem, when will it let me go?"

"Soon … it will let you go soon."

Lisa arrives and sits on Wendy's bed. She puts her arm around her.

"Changing of the guard, Wenz, Hetty can have her cup of coffee now."

"Will you talk with Mum? That's good." She promptly closes her eyes again.

when the time comes for me to die, i know it will be exactly the right time and i will be in the right place. Lately, and it increases all the time, i have been experiencing glimpses and feelings of where i am going. i am going home to unimaginable and indescribable beauty; worlds of universal love, enchanted gardens, sweet music . . . . .

When I get downstairs Janet is teary, a state in which I find her more and more often now.

"Yesterday, when I was sitting next to Wendy on her bed, she opened her eyes, looked at me and said: 'If all the mothers in the world were in the same room, I would always pick you'."

"I said, 'If all the daughters in the world were in the same room, I would always pick you'."

"Then she asked me: 'Even with all the problems I've caused?'"

"And I said to her, 'It's never been a problem. It was, and still is, a magical time, filled with so much love'."

"And then, as if that was not enough, Wendy said, 'When you smile you light up the whole room.' I had a big cry later."

"You know, even with all the tears and pain, we still have moments of laughter. Wendy has never lost her sense of humour. Yesterday Lisa and I were trying to manoeuvre her so we could get her to the toilet. Her nightgown had gone up around her waist and suddenly she said, 'Well, here I am with my pubes exposed for the world to see!' And then she burst out laughing."

A few days later I receive a call from Janet. Wendy's physical condition required an extra dose of steroids in the morning and consequently she became extremely high.

"Wendy was determined 'to go on a trip,' and she ordered Lisa and me to pack her suitcase. We wheeled her around for hours from one bedroom to another, while Wendy decided what had to go in the suitcase — photos, crystals, clothes, special bits and pieces. We first thought she meant the journey, that she might die tonight. It's now 10 o'clock and Lisa and I are exhausted. And Wendy still believes she's going on a trip. Can you please talk to her?"

Janet gives the phone to Wendy. I can hear her breathing.

"Wendy, it's Hetty, I hear you want to go on a trip, but this is not the right time. I want you to wait until you have more strength and then you can go. At this moment I can't allow you to travel. It's not the right time."

I hear her crying. "Wendy, you will go on a trip, but first you need to sleep. Tomorrow morning we'll talk about it again."

Janet calls me back the next morning. Wendy had cried for quite a while but she accepted my decision. This morning when she woke up Wendy wondered why she had all these objects on her bed, and told Lisa and Janet that it was silly to think she'd go on a trip, she was much too sick for that!

Mid-October 1997

WENDY HAS REACHED A STAGE now where she needs continuous help, but with support from her family and visiting nurses this can still be managed at home. Janet and Lisa are constantly adjusting pillows and sheets and rolling her over to alleviate the pain of her bedsores, moistening her lips, putting small blocks of ice in her mouth. She likes her hands and face washed regularly — the cold water cools her down a little.

Rae calls and tells me that Wendy has had severe abdominal pain in the night and is now passing blood and mucus with her motions. We discuss the possibility of internal bleeding. There's nothing we can do but alleviate her pain and try to keep her as comfortable as possible.

I visit Wendy later that day and sit next to her bed. I feel sad and helpless, not being able to relieve her suffering. I watch Janet and Lisa helping, caring, soothing Wendy's aching body, reluctant midwives assisting in the birth of a soul to its final freedom, silently waiting for the final push, the birth, and a new beginning. All through this long and painful labour, Wendy is grateful, thanking people for every act, every deed of kindness.

Friday 17 October 1997

WENDY WAKES UP THIS MORNING in intense pain and discomfort. The family, with the help of Rae and other district nurses, do everything they can to make her more comfortable. Even with the added medication given in her syringe driver and by injection, the pain is relentless and Wendy is getting more and more anxious.

Janet calls me. "She is suffering so much, this can't go on. It can only be a relief for her and everybody when she dies now. She can hardly endure the pain any longer."

Wendy's one plea that morning was "Let me die," and the nurses heard her talking to herself, "Please c'mon, die."

Rae suggests admission to the hospice and Wendy and her family accept. Later that afternoon Wendy leaves her home for the last time. Jessie, her dog, tries to stop the ambulance man, sensing Wendy will not return.

When I arrive at the hospice Wendy is slightly more settled, but still in pain and quite restless. When I bend over her she asks, "Is my room ready?"

I look into her eyes. "Yes, everything is ready for you."

"My room is ready," she murmurs. "My room is ready."

A little later she is given some medication to alleviate her restlessness and increasing discomfort. Together with her family I watch her slowly relaxing, entering a merciful sleep which will carry her to peace within a few hours. Her body finally falling away, releasing the soul to begin its journey home.

In the silence that follows I hear the wind howling outside. Tears are running down my cheeks. Wendy's presence, holding us, lingers in the room.

An experience frozen in time, forever stuck in my memory. It is seven minutes to nine. The sun has set. The night is dark, holding the potential for a new dawn, a new beginning.

I once asked Wendy: "If you could live your life all over again, how would you like it to be different?"

"I would never wish that my life had been any different, because until tonight I've experienced and seen so many special moments, and I know they will continue with the next morning. If I were to wish for differences, then all of those precious pieces wouldn't exist and then I would lose parts of me. Here in me is a flower which blooms with happiness and peace. Love is a chain, once you love one thing, it leads to many others."

A soft rain is falling when I leave the hospice, wetting my face as I look up at the grey and misty sky. Wendy's words reverberate in my mind:

"Once you love one thing, it leads to many others."

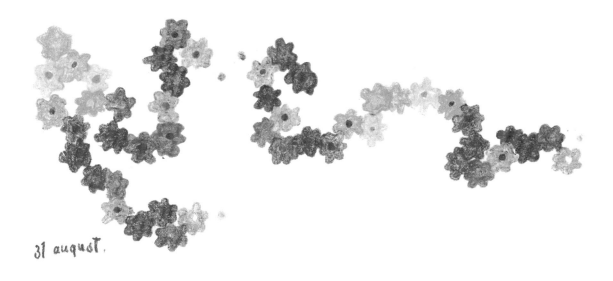

31 august.

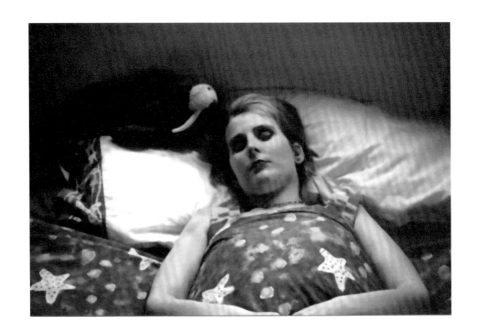

a little finishing letter ...

Inside of me i know that i have finished my work here and that my lesson is learnt. My lesson being that love is the key to every gateway. Love opens to honesty, compassion, respect, understanding, happiness. Love has brought our family, us, so close together, we will never be anywhere but beside one another. And although my time may be very short, in no way is it small.

Medical terms

Biopsy	The removal of tissue from the body for microscopic examination.
Bone marrow	Tissue found at the centre of many long bones of the body. The bone marrow contains stem cells from which all blood cells are made. A sample of these cells is obtained by inserting a needle in the bone, e.g. the sternum or breastbone.
Cervical nodes	Lymphatic glands in the neck area.
Computerised axial tomography (CT scan or cat scan)	A specialised x–ray technique that produces a series of cross-sectional images of the area examined.
Haemoglobin	Protein that carries oxygen in the blood.
Hodgkin's disease	Also known as Hodgkin's Lymphoma. A cancer of the lymphatic system which affects primarily the lymph glands, spleen, and liver.
Inguinal	Affecting the groin.
Lymphadenopathy	Enlarged lymph glands.

Lymphatic system	A vast network of vessels, similar to blood vessels, that branch out into all the tissues of the body. These vessels carry lymph, a colourless watery fluid that carries lymphocytes, specialised white blood cells that protect us against disease and infection. The lymphatic system is part of the body's immune system.
Lymphocyte	Type of white blood cell.
Peripheral stem cell transplantation	Form of cancer treatment where the patient's bone marrow is deliberately destroyed with cancer treatment agents. Immature blood cells (stem cells) are then introduced to the patient in the hope that they will repopulate the destroyed marrow. This might help the bone marrow recover and from then on produce healthy blood cells.
Pulmonary	Referring to the lungs.
Subcutaneous morphine	Battery-operated device that continuously delivers medication through a needle inserted under the skin.
Supra-clavicular fossa	Area above the collarbone.
Shingles	Infection caused by a virus (similar to the chickenpox virus) causing pain and skin eruptions along the course of a particular nerve.

Comments on this book

Caring for people near the end of life can be both rewarding and immensely challenging. In this book Hetty Rodenburg illustrates both of these aspects of care through her compassionate and at times difficult journey in the company of a teenager living with cancer.

I was fortunate to meet Wendy in the latter part of her life and thought I knew something of that story, but what comes through in these pages of narrative, poetry and illustrations is a glimpse into a therapeutic relationship that provides lessons for all who read them.

Starting with some personal reflections on her own 'way of being', Hetty intricately details conversations and events in the last years of this remarkable young woman's life and demonstrates aspects of the true nature of care. Caring is both behaviour and motivation; both are admirably illustrated here.

Wendy touched all who met her with her courage and determination to live right up until the last days of her life. Reading the conversations and watching as the artwork develops over time is both fascinating and at times unsettling. It is a special way of remembering a young woman who touched many lives.

Professor Rod MacLeod
Palliative care physician,
University of Auckland and North Shore Hospice

Hetty came into our life when our 16-year-old son Sam was diagnosed with leukaemia, leaving us all struggling with bewilderment and deep sadness. Her wisdom and loving guidance supported Sam in living his last few years with much joy and happiness, and helped us all to laugh and cry with greater ease.

Wendy's story is one of immense courage and wisdom as she explores pathways and makes choices about her treatment and how she can live with hope and love, whilst preparing to die.

Families facing a similar challenge, seeking answers and wanting to care for their loved one will gain a deeper understanding through this remarkable story. Indeed for anyone diagnosed with a life-threatening illness, I recommend this book.

Alison Bowie
Mother, Wellington

The first time I picked this book up I could not finish it. My 20-year-old son had been through treatment for a very curable cancer and I had a deep emotional response. But like life, there is a time for everything, and when I went back to it, I read it in one sitting and was deeply moved by the love, compassion and humour in the book.

So as a mother and as someone who has been working in hospice for 15 years I recognise that this is an important book for all of us. For health professionals it offers a rare insight in the life and death of a remarkable young woman, and her doctor.

Mary Schumacher
Chief executive, Hospice New Zealand

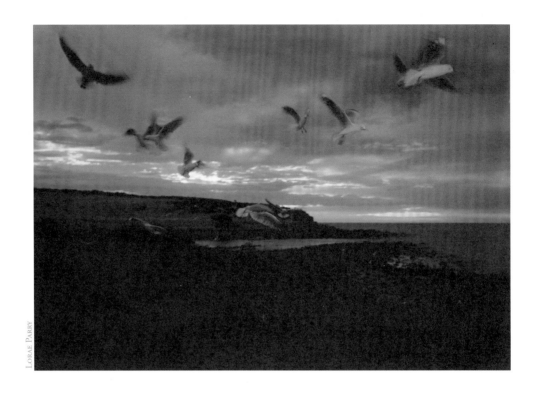

LORAE PARRY

Waste not these few, precious earth years.
The bird of life has but a short arc of time to fly.
Soon — ah, how sadly soon! — it will slip its earthly form
and vanish into the Infinite

Stanza Seven from Moments of Truth —
Excerpts from The Rubaiyat of Omar Khayyam
explained by Paramahansa Yogananda